T0278798

SAVING

A DOCTOR'S STRUGGLE TO HELP HIS CHILDREN

Shane Neilson

GREAT PLAINS
PUBLICATIONS

Great Plains Publications
320 Rosedale Ave
Winnipeg, MB R3L 1L8
www.greatplains.mb.ca

Great Plains Publications gratefully acknowledges the financial support provided for
its publishing program by the Government of Canada through the Canada Book Fund;
the Canada Council for the Arts; the Province of Manitoba through the Book Publishing Tax
Credit and the Book Publisher Marketing Assistance Program; and the Manitoba Arts Council.

"It's Good to Be Here" by Alden Nowlan © Claudine Nowlan, used with permission

Design & Typography by Relish New Brand Experience
Printed in Canada by Friesens

LIBRARY AND ARCHIVES CANADA CATALOGUING IN PUBLICATION

Title: Saving : a doctor's struggle to help his children / Shane Neilson.
Names: Neilson, Shane, 1975- author.
Identifiers: Canadiana (print) 20220496757 | Canadiana (ebook) 20220496781 |
    ISBN 9781773371030 (softcover) | ISBN 9781773371047 (ebook)
Subjects: LCSH: Neilson, Shane, 1975- | LCSH: Neilson, Shane, 1975-—Family. |
    LCSH: Families—Health and hygiene—Canada. | LCSH: Medical care—Canada. |
    LCSH: Neilson, Shane, 1975-—Mental health. | LCSH: Physicians—Canada—
    Biography. | LCGFT: Autobiographies.
Classification: LCC RA418.5.F3 N45 2023 | DDC 613—dc23

ENVIRONMENTAL BENEFITS STATEMENT

Great Plains Publications saved the following
resources by printing the pages of this book on
chlorine free paper made with 100% post-consumer
waste.

TREES	WATER	ENERGY	SOLID WASTE	GREENHOUSE GASES
7	560	3	24	3,030
FULLY GROWN	GALLONS	MILLION BTUs	POUNDS	POUNDS

Environmental impact estimates were made using the Environmental Paper Network
Paper Calculator 4.0. For more information visit www.papercalculator.org

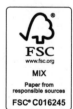

Canadä

FSC
www.fsc.org

MIX

Paper from
responsible sources

FSC® C016245

For Janet, Zee, Kaz, and Conor Kerr

TABLE OF CONTENTS

ENTER BURNING CROWN JESUS

Call it a delusion. Hallucination. Call me crazy.

But I have my very own personal Jesus. He sings to me at night. He howls at the stars, the fire on his golden crown wafting up, sending sparks into the night sky. He sings pornographic hymns—"Gloria" is transformed into "Glory Hole"—and he dances burlesque, shaking his money-maker for tips from the regs. I see him now, waving as if he were an NPC, an avatar. I'm merely waiting to send Jesus on tasks. Go to the neighbour's door and knock, leave a flaming piece of dog poop ignited by the crown. Or knock and not flee, wait for the door to be answered, and have him invite himself in for a cup of coffee. Or walk, instead, down the street, to the convenience store, and bring back a Big Gulp.

My very own personal Jesus prefers the Grape Big Gulps.

The bigger the draught he slurps, the higher his flames rise, the more passionate the hymns, the more suggestive the dancing. He is a trickster God one moment, but then the most loving and appropriate and New Testament-ish heartthrob you could want, a truly sensitive soul who would listen and spoon with me all night. And then other times, a true son of God, the fire and brimstone kind, who recognizes that I have strayed from the true path, that I must get my life right, that, above all, I must not kill myself.

My own personal Jesus has a clipboard now. White coat, thick glasses with thicker frames—the whole deal. He loves visual clichés because he has been represented as a cliché his whole life in Western Civ. He tries on new clichés with aplomb. If there were a visual cliché store, he would shop there.

At the moment, he's decided to be a stock Scientist. He taps the clipboard with a pencil and clears his throat. "Ahem. Ahem ahem." On the page of the clipboard it is written: Thou Shalt Not Die. Commandment numero uno, the first precept in a crazy plan—how to keep Shane alive.

"Why is the commandment only in pencil, Burning Crown Jesus?"

I call him this because, though he has an infinite range of guises and costumes, he is never without the crown. When I have a delusion—meaning, when I believe that someone else is Jesus, that Jesus is something actually happening, something REAL—Jesus is there, perhaps on water skis, a bikini babe on his shoulders, she somehow unsinged by the crown's flames, the crown always perfectly positioned, always secure and unjostled. Perhaps it is his bizarre fashion sense—Elvis Jesus with a burning crown, full Vegas rhinestone, or a straggly sinewy scruffy Woody Guthrie Jesus, a *This Machine Kills Fascists* sticker on the back of a beat-up guitar—that clinches my certainty, an elaborateness to the presentation that simply cannot be faked, the sensory detail required too vast, no mere Photoshop but total green screen. Through it all, the crown is his marker of authenticity, a proof of continuity, a literal article of faith. If there's a burning crown atop a head, then that head is no pretender to the holy throne.

There are times I'm unable to move, experiencing a torpor so profound that it takes me days to exit bed. Psychiatrists call this poverty of movement. Jesus, of course, came from a poor family and lived a life of material poverty, but of great spiritual riches. When I think of the second coming, which I do only rarely, I do not think of an apocalypse. I think of Burning Crown Jesus, on a couch, never moving, catatonically watching Netflix. Time doesn't end; instead, Jesus loses track of the world as the world loses track of itself, humans as distracted as their God.

Amidst this poverty of movement, though, Burning Crown Jesus can, if watched closely for a few hours, ultimately complete a half-turn of his head and mouth the following words:

Thou Shalt Not Die.

"Okay," I say. "I promise, BCJ."

BCJ IS A REFLECTION OF HOW I AM. When Burning Crown Jesus does coke off strippers' tits, or base jumps from a skyscraper, or freebases with a pod of glitter dolphins, or hangs off a bridge by his right arm and tags it with his left, I am being told two things: the first is, I'm high. Not external-chemically, but internal-biochemically. The second message is, of course, God is love. Do I want to put my own personal Jesus at the risk of his personal safety? Moreover, do I want to injure his reputation, his good standing amongst the faithful of the world? When I see BCJ engaging in risky behaviour, I respond in a way I cannot were it reckless me trying to jump from a proverbial diving platform into a bucket of water. I want to say, "Hey, BCJ, it's okay, take it easy. Come over here and let's go get a Gulp. You love Gulp. Let's go Gulp and everything will be cool."

It rarely fails. Jesus can be doing a powdered motorboat and mid-flap, he'll withdraw, slip the lady a twenty in her garter, and walk with me to the 7-11. He might be talking about some crazy stuff, like how he thinks the burning bush is a bit of a Chatty Cathy, or how some day he might like to just take it easy, retire, and live as a demon who possesses people, but only seizes them with an unquenchable desire for flaming hot Cheetos, nothing serious like seizure-convulsions or paralysis or cancer. Jesus can rant and rave on these short walks and I always listen because he always listens to me. We take care of one another. As we reach the clear glass with the painted stripes, the Orange and Green Glade, we call it, the Land O Gulps, Burning Crown Jesus inevitably starts to cry.

"I've strayed from the path laid out for me by the holy father," he says, and the waterworks really flow. But I can always get him out of this state with two things. Sequence is important. We do a material solution first.

"Come inside," I say, "and let's get Gulpy. It's on me." And Jesus is bestowed something greater than incense, frankincense, or myrrh—no sugary sweetness in those. He is gifted with the Grape.

Jesus slurps on the straw. With each little suck, the tears proportionally slow down. His sorrow only plateaus, it doesn't go away, but the Gulp gives him a soothing sensation, it is an act of love.

As we walk back home to the Gulch, where husks of plastic containers litter the floor and fill blue kitchen boxes, all of them pasted with a sticky purple residue, we arrive at not a cathedral or a church but my own room, a small one in a house with a wife and children inside, other creatures that need me and love me but who don't know Jesus, and who can probably never know Him, unless of course they, too, cultivate a similar relationship with their own personal lord and saviour, and may they never need to, may what has and is happening to me never happen to them.

As we walk back, I give him another gift, the spiritual one. I say, "You are saving me, big guy. By straying from the path, you show me the path. You know I love you like a brother, and I fear for you when you are lost. I will always want to walk with you to the Land O Gulps and be there for you."

Now for the tricky part—I have to tell the truth. At least half the time on the walk back home from the Land O Gulps, I realize it is not me talking at all, but Burning Crown Jesus himself; that it is my, not his, face that is wet; that in my hand is a huge goblet of Grape goodness, the glycosylated blood, saturated with more sugar than any adult human male should chug in a year. Half the time, it seems, Burning Crown Jesus is taking care of me and half the time I am taking care of him—the reality of the situation gets confused in my mind—but Commandment numero uno is being respected, honoured, and I remain alive to tell the tale, to you.

BURNING CROWN JESUS IS A WILD MAN. He's turning over chairs, running from one side of the room to the other. "Captain Cavemannnnnnn!" he yells. "Captaiiiiiin Cavemannnnn!"

The Tavern in Cambridge, Rust Belt Ontario, can be a wild spot, but this is a bit much, even for here. I'm not sure I can intervene. BCJ is too hyped up, he can't slow down. How do you reason with someone when they're screaming and running back and forth? Should I tackle him? Throw a drink in his face?

I scream the numero uno, "THOU SHALT NOT DIE," with all my might, but he's unfazed, still playing a manic tag with the walls. Touch, CAPTAIN CAVEMAN. Touch, CAPTAIN CAVEMAN.

The cops will come, I'm sure. BCJ will get thrown into the paddy wagon, locked up, and then sent to the hospital. The doctors will drug him. They will douse his fire according to the rules of the fire marshal as posted in the interior of all public buildings, and then confiscate his crown. He will be left a shell of himself, desecrated, dull. He will not believe any more. Nothing he says will have conviction, only ash remaining of the former flame.

Everyone that used to be in the bar is now out on Grand Street South, watching the crazy straggly-haired unhoused person from the shelter down the road run from one side of the bar to the other, roaring. Everyone except me and Captain Caveman here, who, again, can be distinguished as the Son of God based on the flaming crown that rests on the top of his head, a remarkable headpiece that sits serenely despite the violent flailing of the man, his hurtling. Who is definitely not a straggly-haired street person, that is sacrilege.

If only I had a Big Gulp. If only I could flick a bit of the icy ooze at his face, perhaps the slush would drip into his mouth and he'd have a madeleine moment; or maybe throwing it on the floor would make him slip, and with his movement arrested, he might reflect on how he ended up on his ass, and at that point I could help him up and tell him what they teach us in Critical Incident pedagogy—tell a psychotic assailant I LOVE YOU. It tends to throw them off. Think about it: if you were enmeshed in one of the most distressing moments of your life, what message would you least expect but secretly want the most?

I have no Big Gulp, the Land O is too far away. I need to do something to save the life of my saviour, otherwise I will soon have no future wingman, no celestial bro to save me. What will I do when the first commandment looms in my own life, about to be transgressed, most likely by taking one step off a platform? I can hear the sounds of sirens dopplering their way here. "I love you Burning Crown Jesus!" I yell, bracing myself, closing my eyes, interposing my body between his path and the wall in the centre of the room. I sound like a fan, a groupie.

Rather than getting bodychecked across the bar, I feel instead a strong, confident, manly hug, a whacking-the-back slappy embrace. I open one eye and see a scraggly deity, eyes slightly aglow, crown full blasting, super-hazy flame on. "Hey man," he says. "Don't be sad. Let's go to the Land O Gulps and STAT some Grape. My treat."

"Thanks be to you," I say, in awe.

"And also with you," he says, giving another hearty whack to my back. "Bro."

WHAT IS REAL? In the window, Burning Crown Jesus is seated on a throne, looking bored. Around the throne are clay tablets, rolls of vellum, and several huge vats of grapes. Jesus is a busy man and the tablets and vellum suggest he has much work to do. The grapes are either sustenance or a prelude to a huge future party, hard to know. I wonder if he will invite me to the party. Is this the party?

No. This is official, this is canon, the authoritarian drone of Mr. Big Guy, the energy Old-Testament-inspired even though we are clearly here in audience with Jesus, rock star of the New. The management of this book has decided to speak to you, through me, to provide you with this message. Apparently, there are rules to guide the reader as they move through the loud-quiet-loud grunge of blasphemy in this text. Some points of order must be respected. This is an actual holy sanctum, the real demesne of Jesus, perhaps heaven even, but at the very least one of his legitimate offices.

Yet I can tell, because I know him so deeply, that Jesus is daydreaming. No—strike that. He's not moving. Not at all. Perhaps the spirit has left him. Perhaps this is only a statue with a burning crown, an icon of an icon. "Sire, you have visitors," I say, hoping that this stimulus is enough to capture his attention.

BCJ suddenly stands, as if an automaton. His mouth opens and closes in a rhythmic fashion while a tinny recording plays from somewhere in his midsection. The sound dubbing is comically poor, as if a Japanese anime (Voltron, maybe?) were playing behind an audio discoursing about mint juleps in the month of May as voiced in a southern drawl, perhaps by Delta Burke.

For your reading pleasure, this is an Enter Burning Crown Jesus production. In this text, you will hear of strange doings in the night. There will be improbable beasts! Sacrilege. Thrills and chills! You will hear a doctor tell-ing tales out of school. He will speak of system and disappointment! And so much crying about his children!

To the left of this simulacrum of BCJ, a different speaker sounds: *BOOOO. HISSSS!*

Back to belly-of-tin-Jesus-speaker: *Children will be maimed in this text, they will almost die! Beware! The vassal writing these lines for you now will have his heart broken over and over again, for this is, above everything else, a love story. Really, I'm a bit of a sadist. I insist on a quota of broken hearts, it's good for the salvation business. Now put your hands inside the ride and keep them there at all times! And don't you dare forget to leave a Google review!*

The automaton jerks back to its sitting position, mouth continuing to spasm open and closed for a few more seconds until it, too, stops. A sound comes from a hidden speaker on BCJ's right: *Come, sit at my right hand.*

There is no place to sit, though. Tablets and vellum crowd the space. Luckily, a small portal opens in one of the vats, showing a screen. There, saying *Cha Cha Cha Cha* and waving jazz hands, is BCJ himself, the real one, the one I know and love. He's wearing a red smoking robe.

"Shane, this part is for you. Not for the audience. You know I'm always there for you, right?"

"Yes, Jesus. Why do you look like Hugh Hefner today?"

"Do I look like Hef? I thought I was just getting my comfort on, you know? I'm trying something new, trying to be just good enough. Just good enough for today. I'm not sure people will like it—the faithful. They tend to like the all-powerful version, the dude with intercessions, thunderbolts and lightning, the laying on of hands. That dude is classy. But lately, it's like maybe I can just be good enough for one day. Wear silk pajamas and hit the grotto. Maybe, at the end of the day, I'll say to myself: today was a good day! Anyway, that's what I'm hoping."

"Maybe the original sin of religion was the idea of perfection itself."

"Yeah, bro. You get it! You get *me*. So *philosophical*, dude! But there is something I want to get right today. Just one thing I want to get per-fect. Old habits die hard I guess. Or at least, old habits die hard until the third day, and then they rise again! Hahahaha!"

Jesus, with his dad jokes. "What's that, BCJ?"

"I want us to have the talk," BCJ says.

"What talk? You and I are in constant communication. We regularly review the first commandment."

"No, no, not that. The talk about reception," BCJ says. "I'm always engaged in this PR stuff. Big Christianity is obsessed with optics. So I have a little experience in this regard."

"What regard?"

"Well, you know what they'll say about your book," says Burning Crown Jesus.

"I know," I say. "What they always do."

BCJ raises his right eyebrow. The right eyebrow of the Son of God. Somewhere on the earth, a hurricane is getting ginned up by divine action.

I shrug. "Who cares about those people. They never cared."

"You know," BCJ says, eyebrow down. He's serene again. "You *know*," he adds, nodding for emphasis.

He's so real. He *is* real, even though his likeness is beaming from a television screen. I love him and he loves me. He never offers advice. His presence *is* advice. It's a warning. A loving warning, a signal to not let go, to stay alive. To keep faith. The flames from his crown lick perfection but never taste it, only the crack in all our souls, our faithless moment or moments on the cross. Lick, lick, lick. As they undulate, they cast a warm light.

"I know you don't care, Shane. I know you want to help the world, to make these things okay to talk about. I know you think that telling this story will help your family and other families, that you shouldn't be ashamed to tell the story, that there's nothing shameful about it. And I agree with you."

"So why are you asking?"

"I'm not sure you know about the cost."

BCJ knows about cost. He was crucified, died, and was buried. He knows I'm listening, that I always listen to him. And that's enough for both of us. It's our deal.

"I've thought this through," I respond. "They'll say I shouldn't say anything. That a physician doesn't tell secrets about his kind. They might use my admissions of personal illness against me. And they'll also say, more than anything, that I am not allowed to be honest when I write about my children. They'll turn that honesty around and bully me with it, just as they bullied me when I was a child."

BCJ smiles. The thick red robe does not singe even though, as a game, BCJ pulls the robe over his eyes, then drops it, mouthing *peekaboo peekaboo*. The robe brushes against his crown. I've always wanted to reach up and warm my hands by that fire, see how hot it is, but I never have, held back by the worry that the gesture would be somehow disrespectful.

"You know if that happens, I will always be here for you."

"Yes, I know."

This is a variation on our standard goodbye. BCJ says he will always be there, and as per the ritual, I acknowledge the fact. All these years, it's been enough to keep me alive.

"Good luck," he says, his face wet, the tears sizzling as they run down his cheeks.

"You're not leaving, are you?" I ask.

"Oh no. You know that I'll always be with you."

A LOVE STORY

Burning Crown Jesus walks into traffic. Burning Crown Jesus climbs the rungs of a water tower, nearly reaching the top, waving at me as he steps over the last rung. Burning Crown Jesus jumps from a moving bus and is smucked by a garbage truck. Burning Crown Jesus sticks a fork into an electric socket. Burning Crown Jesus slips a noose around his neck, ties the rope to an overhead beam, then steps off the chair. Burning Crown Jesus pours kerosene on himself and lights a match. Burning Crown Jesus sticks his head into a gas oven. Burning Crown Jesus goes to the pawn shop downtown and purchases a shotgun. Since they don't have shells, he picks some up at Canadian Tire. He loads the shotgun and puts the barrel in his mouth. Burning Crown Jesus pulls a knife from the drawer and tries to cut off his head. Burning Crown Jesus jumps into the polar bear pen at the Toronto Zoo.

"Shane, I said I would die for you. But this is ridiculous, don't you think?" By my count, BCJ has died over fifty times today, and he may need to die many more yet.

"I'm sorry, BCJ. Maybe it's time to go to the Land O Gulps. I think I owe you this time."

Slowly, we walk, BCJ's right leg dragging behind him, blood spurting from every gashed limb, an inexhaustible supply. "Jesus, heal thyself," I say.

As soon as he's back in perfect shape, though, his eyes once more in his head and his skull not crushed, I see that he's gazing at the road, ruminating about whether to take another step into traffic.

FOR THE SUICIDAL, a single method is eventually settled upon and soon becomes the focus of their attention.

Suicidology is an academic discipline of recent advent, originating in the mid-twentieth century. The "father of suicidology," Edwin Shneidman, defines suicide as "a conscious act of self-induced annihilation, best understood as a multidimensional malaise in a needful individual who defines an issue for which the suicide is perceived as the best solution." Despite definition, which in this case seems quite satisfactory to me, the discipline cannot, at bottom, explain the mystery by answering the question of *why*. Here, risk factors and psychological autopsies of personal circumstances are misleading. A resultant false story, tidy enough to understand, forms to make survivors feel better in the aftermath of a suicide.

A question incompletely answered is one families find less unsettling than a complete mystery. The most material answer—sometimes the only one possible—is how the suicide was accomplished. Methods are concrete. They distract attention away from the mystery of the act—*Why?*—to the much easier question of *How?* Method is tactile whereas why is convoluted, fractured, invisible thought.

To show you the why, I'm writing to you now. I'm telling you the story.

THIS IS A LOVE STORY. It starts with a knock at the apartment door—through the eyehole I see Janet, the master's student I met at a bar just a few weeks ago. I'm twenty-three years old, and not like many other people. I never have been like other people, but I'm not conscious of that yet. At the same time, difference is something I feel, something I've always felt.

A few hours earlier, the sun had set and I, as per rigid routine, had watched it go down from my twentieth-floor apartment balcony. In the dark, I am social with all the other impermanent little lives turning lights on and off in adjacent apartment buildings, pocket suns going nova and then snuffing out. Person there, person no longer there.

At some point, there are too few lit windows to sustain a community vigil. Lists flit through my mind to make me feel somehow both less alone and more anxious. Drug management of congestive heart failure:

carvedilol; furosemide; nitroglycerin drip; spironolactone. The major criteria of Rheumatic Fever: Syndenham's chorea; erythema marginatum; myocarditis; subcutaneous nodules; polyarthritis. The ACLS drug protocol for ventricular tachycardia: epinephrine; amiodarone; lidocaine. Lists sing and soothe, are rungs on a ladder that exercise my mind, are poetry. My memory is my friend, a self-administered treatment for aloneness.

Through the eyehole, I see Janet sway. She reaches out her left arm to stabilize. When I open it, she lists into me, pulls at my belt, leading me to a bed she'd never been in before. "The intercom has your name written next to your apartment number. 'prise!"

One time we chatted on College Street. I was leaving the building late at night; she was going in. "I prefer to do my work in the lab when no one's there," she said. "I like the quiet, the focus."

This I could really understand. The late evening was cold, the kind of fall day in Halifax when sunny mornings were comfortable in a T-shirt, but nightfall made the previous warmth seem as if it happened somewhere else. "I'm just going home," I said, wearing an off-white X-Men T-shirt with Cyclops bursting out in front of Rogue, Wolverine, and Gambit, his red energy beam destroying something out of the frame.

"Is it far?" she responded, in a turquoise ski jacket.

"No. It's just over there, on Spring Garden. See the ground floor? The oldies are still checking their mailboxes." And you *could* see: bland shapes moving slowly from the elevator to a large grey wall and back, olds who hoped for letters from other olds.

Janet wriggles out of her jeans and straddles me. I've always been curious about difference. Smart and small, she seems quirky. She hits against me as hard as she can, and though I'm coming, I'm also remembering, too, a list of places we've visited together in the past two weeks: a German language class offered at a festival down by the docks; the T-Room, watering hole for blotto engineers, lights low perpetually and on purpose; brief chats in the Tupper Building lobby, light showering through big bay windows; a recital of the Tupper Concert band, Janet as first clarinet, hair left down and long. She falls to the left side of the bed, the side she's taken ever since.

"I came here straight from The Lower Deck," she said. From open to close, the Lower D offers an idiot mix of dance pop and Stan Rogers. I had danced with other girls there before, watched groups of young men throw their arms around one another and bray "Barrett's Privateers." Everyone brayed, it was a thing and remains a thing. "I went out with the lab girls. But it was depressing," she said.

"Why did you find it depressing?"

"Ugh. So many sailors. So many men with tan lines on their ring fingers." To me, this sounded very worldly. My mating strategy so far was to not have one, to simply be kind. But then to advertise this as a "mating strategy" would perhaps reveal the nature of the problem.

"I realized I could stay there and meet someone, also drunk, and go home with them. Or I could come to you, someone who was genuine. Who really liked me."

"Was it worth it?" I asked.

"Remains to be seen," she said.

Hmmmph.

"Did you sing Barrett's Privateers?" I asked before she fell asleep.

"Yeah, I joined in on the chorus. Isn't it, like, a Halifax bylaw?"

Lists dissipated in my mind like a drunken man on a Halifax pier. For once, I joined the darkness outside the window and fell asleep.

AT AGE TWENTY-SEVEN, I had been practising medicine for over two years as a resident doctor. Most of those days, I wanted to die. Each night I wasn't working in the hospital, I descended the staircase leading to the street exit of our upper-level apartment. In a small nook, I wrote a series of poems about the neglect and abuse I suffered as a child. I tried to make the pain as beautiful and concentrated as I could. But something went wrong along the way—each descent a deepening of the meaning, a more intense concentration of the events until, somehow, the pain seemed inevitable, permanent, permeating, until there was just one more link to build in that chain, a few more steps to take.

The night that the poems felt like they were completed, that there was nothing to change or add, I wrote a goodbye letter to my wife, explaining that she didn't do anything wrong. If there was a reason I had to die, I neglected to inform her. Perhaps the poems, if she ever found them, would explain. Maybe BCJ would come to her, too, and reveal that it was part of some bullshit plan, that he had done the best he could, had reminded me of the numero uno, but I just wouldn't listen.

I climbed the stairs, wondering if I should look in on my wife and daughter as they slept one last time. But if I looked in on them, my reasoning went, I might stop. There might be no end to the mystery.

Burning Crown Jesus stared out of the laptop screen as I wrote the final poem. "Shane, I have been watching over you, and I'm going to tell you our secret code so that you know it's me. I'm not a false hallucination or something your brain is tricking you with so that you'll abandon the plan. Remember the failsafe we rehearsed, our safety protocol?"

Many years ago, BCJ and I developed a last-ditch mechanism in case I become so unwell that I am in too great a danger of suicide. We worked on it so that any false hallucination would fail to come up with the correct codeword. I would never tell any other part of my brain, or anyone else, and we both knew that BCJ would never tell another soul, living or dead. "Okay, Burning Crown Jesus," I said. "Let's see if you're the real Burning Crown Jesus. What's the safe word?"

BCJ was unfazed. He peered at me as his flames maintained their perpetual vigilance. Staring contest. Okay. I blinked 1,202 times at the small blaze roiling above BCJ's head. He never blinked. After my 1,202 defeats, I realize: the safe word was no word. The safe word was more of an act: just watching.

"Okay. We've proved that we're real to one another," said Burning Crown Jesus.

"Fine. You're real, Burning Crown Jesus," I admitted.

I recalled his face on the cross, a static agony depicted in countless Catholic crucifixion scenes. Christ in pain; Christ not wanting to be in pain; Christ as human; Christ as, somehow, the son of God.

"I have appeared unto you," he said.

"I know."

"Then you know what this means," he said.

"I know."

What does life mean? How is life possible? I didn't ask.

"Please," he said, because there was no longer anything he could do.

Janet must have heard me open the heavy sliding door to the balcony, for I was no longer alone. The glass door behind me slid open with a shout.

"Shane! No! Commandment numero uno!"

But I was balanced on the ledge, already over the railing. From where I stood, I could see Halifax slope towards the harbour, the windows of houses tinted with light. So many people still awake. The occasional car ambled down the street.

I looked back past Janet to the sliding window. What I'm writing now might not be true. I suffered a head injury and my memory of the incident isn't perfect. And Janet disputes this. But what I remember is sometimes brought forward to me in the present when I look at a window. I see a three-year-old girl with blond ringlets. Little Zee. She must have been woken up from her midnight snuggle session by the motion of her mom. She's wearing a fuzzy onesie, and her head is pressed against the glass.

I jump.

WAKE. THE SHEETS SLOWLY RISE AND FALL over a slender, hourglass outline that silhouettes the window's morning light, partially obstructing my view of the harbour. The window is where my mind always goes. If I change the routine, then my whole life will collapse. My brain works like this. Above the woman's small body, a plume of smoke ascends from the assisted-living high-rise opposite. The visual effect is that the woman in front of me is burning.

What the hell happened? A black-haired, tiny, naked, half-Japanese scientist gently snores beside me. The routine regime dictates that I glance between buildings to gauge shadow so as to determine time of day. I can tell from the visible sky that the time is somewhere between 5:30 and 6 AM but between-building gap light specifies more precisely. Janet's form, though, blocks those gaps. Or fills them in? Routines are rigid, unbreakable. My waking one has been the same for as long as I can remember. To deviate from a routine is to feel a sense of impending doom in the form of a stake impaling the chest. But these are just thoughts, they are not that feeling. Maybe I am happy. In what becomes a new ritual easily replacing its predecessor, I reach around Janet's small waist to spoon and fall asleep again, but not before comparing the light outside the window to mist.

SOMETIMES GROWTH OCCURS IN NEGATIVE TERMS. Sometimes, growth is *in* and not *out, down* and not *up*. Paradoxical growth: how darkness expands so that we learn what we really are. The cause of this growth comes from constantly approaching the world to receive the same feedback: *you are not wanted, you are not necessary, you are a problem*. Pain is the signal of discordance, of a discrepancy between self-concept and reality.

One secret of faith I've learned under the watchful eyes of BCJ: there is no quantifying of belief, and no number to apply to abstraction. BCJ was not asked what his pain was like on a scale of one to ten when he was nailed to the cross. His suffering was incalculable. Comparing miseries is the illness of the Philistines.

IN THE PUBLIC GARDENS, platoons of male ducks serially hold their mates down, bite their necks and sit on their backs. A few seconds later, they convulse, and then release their females. The males stand still, unwilling to give any ground. The females ruffle their feathers back into a semblance of decorum and dart away as other ducks watch from the shade of a tree or bush.

As the spring wears on, more of the park shrubbery becomes home for mothers with chicks. If any young park patron steps toward a nest, the mother becomes erect; take another step and she puffs more, making a clicking sound; another step and she emits an aggrieved squawk. Just a month before these birds would run in fear should a toddler chase them. Now they would fight to the death if an interloper moved toward their young.

At twenty-four, I had seen over a hundred mothers give birth on the obstetrics floor of the Grace, that pinky-bluish hospital tucked off Summer Street. None of those women seemed like Janet. In the main, they were older, in their thirties. Janet seemed physically more substantial to me, even though the new mothers were literally creating human substance. Janet felt denser, harder, heavier, somehow less generic. And now she is unexpectedly pregnant with our child. Halifax has given me a new estimation of fatherhood.

I link my arms behind Janet's back and pull her into me. "How are you?"

"I'm vomiting still in the mornings. And I sleep more now." She rolls over. Visible just above her backside are two completed pregnancy tests on the dresser from the night before. Four blue stripes.

"What are we going to do?" I ask.

YESTERDAY, I WORKED AS A DOCTOR IN THIS PLACE. I wore a white coat. Now I'm on a gurney in the major trauma section.

Dr. James was born in a white coat. He goes to sleep in a white coat. Not once in my life have I seen him without a white coat on his back. I think James was born in England based on a vestigial accent, there's a natal Britishness about him. But who knows. These kinds of thing you can't just ask: *Hey dude, what's with the accent? Hey man, are you glued into that white coat?*

At any rate, I decided to like James a long time ago, after he took care of an old drunk man with chronic subdural hemorrhages. After the neurosurgeon came and recommended burr holes, the confused man kept bawling in his bed. Nurses gave the man tablet after tablet of lorazepam, enough to make a whole ward of patients unmoor.

James, though, had curiosity. He went behind the curtain and talked to the old man, who, as it turns out, had a cat. James dialed the old man's next of kin, who was really his neighbour since his family had fled long ago, and asked the neighbour to feed the old man's cat. He listened as the old man painstakingly explained just how much food to put out and on what kitchen shelf it was stored.

James: a 'People Who Care.' A People Who Care is a term from my secret clinical lexicon, an honorific that designates paid health care staff—be they physician, physician assistant, nurse, occupational therapist, physiotherapist, social worker, or radiation technologist—who connect with patients and families despite a bureaucracy designed to crush their souls, to take advantage of their goodness by exploiting it as capital. Rather than depersonalize in the face of endless, impossible work, they find meaning in that work despite the odds. People Who Care is a term both singular and plural. People Who Care is a divine element in an otherwise uncaring system. People Who Care can't redeem that system, but they make it a little more tolerable. They make grief and loss sear and scar a little less.

I blurt out something important that James needs to know. "You need to call the army, James! The Germans are about to mount an assault on Halifax." I point to someplace beyond the department's eastern wall, to where I think the harbor should be. "They're going to come by sea."

James turns to the nurses who are getting me settled. "Let radiology know we need an urgent CT head." At first, I think this funny—James has good comedic timing, stemming perhaps from a life lived in affectation. But then I realize he's serious. He shines a penlight into my eyes and checks my reflexes with an orange-topped rubber hammer. "Tell radiology he's GCS 14 because his best verbal response is confused."

What? I'm not confused. The Germans are coming. Canada is under attack. Patriots, answer the call!

"Damn, Shane, what happened?" he asks.

I really don't know, either. I walked up some stairs? I can't remember much after that. But this I know: the Germans are coming.

Someone incessantly vomits nearby, unable to reset the nausea program. Despite Olympic retching, nothing's ejected for minutes. Monitors make unsynchronized alarms, the beeps clambering over one another. Gurneys bang against the walls of the central nursing area as paramedics wheel in different acuities of our collective human drama. And yet the place possesses the quality of quiet somehow, as if all noise is private, as if one is eavesdropping. All the misery here is both reluctantly sole-sourced and collective.

Like all emergency departments everywhere, there are no windows. Without them, my insularity cannot escape itself. I can't think linearly if there is no vector for thought, no place for it to go, only space for swirl.

James is still standing there, waiting for an answer. How long has he been standing there? What does he see?

"The Germans are coming... ."

"WHAT DO YOU WANT TO DO?" she asks back, and it sounds like there's just curiosity there, no defined opinion, no demand. Mostly, I don't know what she thinks, which is why I can fall asleep next to her. Two bodies thinking at my habitual velocity could power a city. One body thinking can pour its thoughts into the other dark body and simply fall asleep.

Fate is the ultimate arbiter—political positions and personal convictions do not count for much. The most honest answer I could give Janet is, *I want to be with you*. I know I want to keep this chance, I have nothing else.

On my apartment shelves are hardcover first editions by Alden Nowlan, books of poems that contain their own discourse on love, how it is something that is desperate, choked, or never said aloud. These poems seem closest to my own concept of love, a thrum deep within that is difficult to believe in, but which yet resounds through all life.

There has never been a time when what I will say matters so much. I think of Nowlan's "It's Good to Be Here," an imagined dialogue between his parents as they decided what to do about his conception out of wedlock:

> Then she cried and then
> for a long time neither of them
> said anything at all and then
> their voices kept rising until
> they were screaming at each other
> and then there was another long silence and then
> they began to talk very quietly and at last he said
> well, I guess we'll just have to make the best of it.
> While I lay curled up,
> my heart beating,
> in the darkness inside her.

As a student, I've watched couples' faces during discussions about fertility with reproductive specialists. They are desperate to hear good news, their faces form the expression that *Please* makes—an expression held for an entire twenty minutes. Should I orate to Janet about building a family that loves one another, a better family than the one I had been born into?

I don't know what I'm doing or thinking. I feel my thoughts accelerate and yet not fracture; they shove themselves out to the window. Somehow, I'm not thinking anymore. The window and my mind are continuous. I say, "When I go to other people's houses, I often play with the children. It's more fun. I think I understand them better."

Though I've watched the savviest of doctors discoursing to their patients about uncertainty, dispensing reassurance as if it were an actual treatment, *this* is the most persuasive I can be? We don't say anything for a while. I put my hand on Janet's belly and hold it there. My thoughts return, albeit much slower, as a series of images that concern broken and derelict things dredged from my own history: a Christmas tree with a tinfoil star on top, a daddy longlegs trapped under a bucket, a sleep blanket torn to shreds. Rather than stream to the window, they trickle down my neck and arm, into her normal-sized belly. Is the life of a child a decision one can make according to the logic of poetry?

Yes? Poetry is for emotion. No? This decision requires reason. Resorting to prose, I say something practical: "I want the baby, but I'll support your decision either way. If you keep the baby, and we don't stay together, I promise to be the baby's father." Why not just say, *I want to be with you?* That seems germane. "I'll be a good father," I add, my face adopting the *Please* formation, but not for her—for myself.

"I'm glad you're here," she says, putting her hand on my hand. As usual, Janet says the important thing, the thing I wanted to say. I undress, climb on top of her, and we say nothing more for a while more.

IN A SMALL ROOM ADJACENT TO THE DEPARTMENT, Dr. Black asks me all the things I have also asked suicidal patients after unsuccessful attempts.

1. "Why did you jump off the balcony?"
   I'm not sure. But I'll never do it again. Please let me go.

2. "How long have you been feeling this way?"
   Not long?

3. "If we were to discharge you now, what would you do?
   I would be good.

4. "What would keep you from trying to die again?"
   My wife. My daughter.

Every answer is, of course, lies. I know what happens to people who tell the truth in this situation. If I told Dr. Black that dying is my destiny, that it has always been, that I will jump from the MacDonald Bridge after he lets me out of here, that there is nothing that can stop me from dying, what else could he do, but lock me up?

Dr. Black is still talking, but since he's not asking questions, I don't listen. Inside my head, this anthem blares: *Let me go let me go let me go.* Except the anthem is leaking outside. Dr. Black is staring like BCJ stares. I realize I am whispering the anthem again and again.

Dr. Black didn't need to interview me at all. James might as well have written in the disposition section of the chart, "FUCKING ADMIT THIS GUY OTHERWISE HE WILL THROW HIMSELF UNDER A BUS FIVE MINUTES AFTER DISCHARGE."

Wrong. I will jump from a bridge. Faithless fool.

I want to tell Dr. Black about the Germans because he, too, seems like a People Who Care. I want to save him if he will be saved, if he will listen. But how can I die if I tell him about the Germans? Maybe he will think I'm crazy. James thought I was crazy. Now feels like a bad time to talk about them. So, I stick to the script, say nothing. I try to look normal, though that's never worked before, not once, no passing for me, just passing strange. I will tell Dr. Black about the Germans at the last minute, when he needs to be saved.

"You know, you could have died," Dr. Black says, matter-of-factly.

When was the last time Dr. Black wore a white coat? A V-neck black sweater overlays a dark blue dress shirt, the upper third of a bright red tie erupting on his chest. Thank god he is not wearing a bowtie—the surest sign of a medical prick. The irony of psychiatry is that the suicide of patients is always a practitioner's singular, greatest fear, and yet the shrinks never have to professionally deal in blood.

What to say to Dr. Black? A strategy comes into view: admit to the crime and see if the copper will let me go. "I think that was the point," I say. Mustering up sincerity, a quality that should never require mustering, I say, "But I don't feel that way now."

I do, though. I try to present myself as professionally as possible, answering his questions with the respect due a superior. Imagine: near the end, wanting to be dead, I still want to be perceived as a good student. I am good. Perfection is the original sin, encasing all our fates, none of us agreeing that we are good enough, that we *are* good.

Dr. Black asks his questions with genuine compassion. He doesn't do the quick version for a foregone admission, as I have done in the past in the interests of efficiency, of expediency, of not picking the scab. I am as obvious an admission as they come, but Dr. Black shows curiosity, gently expressing concern.

Luckily, I am so sick that the truth is displayed right on my face, my posture, tone, and expressions all contradicting the content of my speech. Words are one thing, but being in the same room with someone is another. They have an energy. And sometimes, they are filled to the brim with a death-wish. To wit: let me die, stop wasting my time. Let me satisfy this need. I am good, but I need to get good and gone.

"I think you need to stay with us, Shane. It sounds like you very much want to go home and that is commendable, but it just isn't safe to let you go home right now, and we will evaluate this situation over the coming days. We want to make sure that you feel good."

Stay with us. He says this so nicely, so reasonably, that I can't object. Nor would I object. He is my superior. And he needs saving too, he just doesn't know it yet. And I am good. I do not feel good. There is a difference.

"WHAT NAMES ARE YOU THINKING OF?" Janet asks. I don't know. I'm thinking of inapplicable names, biblical names, ones doomed to be laughed at. Who among us wants to be named Zebulon? As if an asteroid had just impacted the earth in front of me from outer space—who knows how long I'm lost to thought, really, the duration feels infinite—Janet says, "I want the girl's name to be Zdeňka."

"You want *what?*"

"I want the name, if she's born a girl, to be Zdeňka."

"What?" I say again.

"*ZDEHNGKAH*," she says, slowly and clearly.

I say, "Stenka."

"No. Zdeňka."

"Za-denka."

"No. Try to do *JJJJJ* at the start. *JJJJJ.*"

"Zdenka."

"Okay, better. But don't forget the grapheme."

"What?"

"Grapheme—oh, never mind. You've got it except for the ň. ŇŇŇŇŇŇŇŇŇ!" Janet now makes the proper n noise, which in technical terms is the palatal nasal.

Zebulon Zebulon Zebulon.

I say my daughter's name properly for the first time, on the fifth try: "Zdeňka."

"Yes!" Janet says. "You got it!"

A year before we met, Janet spent time in Hradec-Králové of the newly-formed Czech Republic. She studied in the Faculty of Medicine Building there, a structure that from the outside looks like a restoration of the Roman Coliseum. Running around that country are a platoon of Zdeňkas and Zdeňeks, and she thought the female form very beautiful.

A strange name to Canadian ears, Zdeňka will be doomed to perpetual mispronunciation and a further confusion stemming from Janet's visible ethnicity. What is the difference between the oddness of Zebulon and Zdeňka? If anything, Zdeňka is harder to pronounce. The child will experience serial mispronunciations during roll calls of various kinds—school. Girl guide camps. Every official interaction involving a checking of ID. Police. Receptionists.

But. Her name will also be unusual, special, distinctive. Plus, her nickname will be Zee—the best letter in the alphabet, no contest, my all-time favourite. Perhaps Zebulon and Zdeňka are equivalent in this way, destined to drop into the letter shorthand.

Zee Zee Zee.

In 2000, the top birth names for Canadian girls were Emily, Madison, Olivia, Hannah, Abigail, Isabella, Samantha, Elizabeth, and Ashley. Zdeňka vaults over those mean-girl names, bouncing on their vowelly softness. Zee is beautiful.

AN ORDERLY I DON'T KNOW inserts a key into the number panel, then presses a button. The spacious elevator—no doubt this large to comfortably transport patients strapped to their beds—takes me up to the eighth floor of the Abbie Lane building. Mr. Orderly is my escort, ensuring I don't elope. Our gentleman's agreement is that I won't. I like that the elevator is going up, that direction definitely has potential.

I contemplate bolting once the elevator doors open, finding a set of stairs, then making my way to the MacDonald Bridge. Whenever I've crossed it by car, travelling to the Dartmouth General Hospital, I've noted the sidewalk and longingly looked to the water forty-seven metres down, the sun too bright to look directly below, the seawater a radiant apocalypse.

Let's jump together, Mr. Orderly, you and I, the evening spread out against the sky like dead men on the mortuary table. Let us go, beside a crowded freeway, hands interlaced as terminal lovers, one final date and destination, the water with a density of 997 kg/m^3, we can accompany one another to the crushed and impacted vale, you can truly learn what it is to escort another and I can know what it means to be free, finally, the freest of free, in complete free-fall.

The elevator door opens, but escape is futile. Entry to the ward is controlled. For starters, no stairwell. The space between the elevator and wall opposite is just big enough for a bed. The only way out of this enclosure is back by elevator or forward through a heavy metal door that leads into the ward.

Waiting for me on the other side of the door is a displaced voice piped in by intercom. A female voice. She says, "We need your shoes." Her intonation is distinctly that of command.

Meahh.

Quite reasonably, I say to the voice, "No. I need my shoes. How am I supposed to walk in the hospital? There could be VRE. MRSA."

"That's the protocol," she says. "You'll get them back when we think you're well enough."

Oh.

"The door to the ward is locked, you need to get buzzed through one and then another. You need to have privileges to leave. I'm telling you this so that you know. You'll see when we bring you in." Meaning: I'm telling you this so that you don't try to escape.

The elevator door closes. I remember that it works by key. Behind me, I don't hear the rustle of Mr. Orderly's greens. Nevertheless, I feel him move closer.

I wish Dr. Black were here. I'd do as *he* asked. But not because he is my superior. Because he is a People Who Care. With no other option except a poor one—and I've never struck another human in my life—I slip off my shoes. My red-stockinged feet make for a ridiculous contrast against the off-white linoleum floor.

"Now for sharps. Do you have any?"

Sensing my confusion—is there a camera here?—she asks, "Do you have any knives, or objects with sharp edges?"

I don't, but Mr. Orderly conducts an inspection nevertheless to verify the fact. I'm right—he was closer. I'm not patted down, but my pockets are emptied to ensure I have no syringes or blades.

"We get all kinds in here," the voice says.

"I know," I say. I think this funny, and laugh. The voice of Mr. Orderly doesn't. For me, this feels like an abandon-hope-all-ye-who-enter-here moment. For them, it's protocol.

Mr. Orderly makes a thumbs up sign. "Go through the door now," the voice commands.

A long hallway extends and then opens up to the right, where a nurses' station gazes on a nest of rooms. I look back and see a black and white screen display showing Mr. Orderly soundlessly disappear into the elevator. Why aren't any of the ward doors closed? Oh. Right.

The voice, now attached to a middle-aged nurse in street clothes, deposits me in a room meant for two people, but there's no other occupant. My red socks are incredible suns, the most alive thing to be found at floor-level.

A ward clerk appears. He's big, slow-moving, and surly. My socks are much more alive than he is. I sense he is not a People Who Care. "Your wife brought you this," he says, shoving a plastic bag at me. Then he turns around like a tank and treads away.

"Can I see her?" I ask his back.

"She left the package at the Emergency Department," he says on his way out the door. "She can't come up here."

I watch him return to the nurses' station to sit in an office chair larger than all the rest. Three nurses at the station laugh together in conversation, but he's frowning at a computer terminal. Something on the screen is angrifying. Perhaps an annoying duck just sent him an email asking him for grapes.

I walk back to my bed and look inside the plastic bag, the universe constricting to the size of a loaded shaving razor with three spare blades in a transparent package. Janet brought me my toothbrush and shaving kit. The glint mesmerizes until I notice a fractionated face shrunk to blade-size, just eyes and crown visible. BCJ.

"Are you sure you want to do this, Shane?"

"Burning Crown Jesus, I haven't seen you in a long, long time. I wondered if you had forgotten about me. Or if I wasn't worth visiting anymore."

"You know I am always with you, Shane. I am always here, always waiting."

BCJ's fiery top is eerie in the reflected brightness. He seems sicklier, more like me.

"I must die," I tell him.

Against type, BCJ sounds pissed. Flames crackle above his head. "Shane, what has feeling ever done for you in your life? What has it ever proven or shown you? How important is it when you forget what it felt like just a few days later? How often have the decisions taken just a few days before seemed impulsive and illogical?"

BCJ never tells me what to do. He only listens. I close my eyes to dissipate the slight hiss from his flames, like letting air from a tire. When the sound is completely gone, I open them. BCJ has disappeared from the silver metal. From down the hallway, a duck completes his bow-tied transformation into J. Alfred Prufrock, daring to disturb the universe, knowing that there is time for decisions that will reverse.

I set to work on my left wrist, pulling, pushing, and ripping, trying to get at my radial artery. Five minutes later, the blood's not flowing heavily enough and the macerated tissue obscures the vessel, though I feel it deep below. My wrist is shredded but I'm not dying quickly.

I move up to the left antecubital fossa to expose the brachial artery. I dissect myself, moving the blade more carefully, sequentially moving through successive layers: epidermis, dermis, fascia. The pulsing, pinkish structure soon comes into view. I touch it and watch the artery slightly recoil. Blood splashes the bedsheets.

The vessel is alive, a red and living thing, just like my socks. It is like the sun, the eternal moment of my greatness flickering, Prufrock about to perfect himself, finally achieving his dream to become Hamlet.

The ward clerk returns. "What the hell?" He yells out, "Code White! Code White!"

The slumbering ward comes alive. Someone slaps the blade out of my hand.

When I wake up, simple interrupted sutures blossom on my wrist and elbow. I don't know where I am. The room is bare, the floors and walls soft, a single heavy door the only exit. I can't use my arms to lift myself up, they're too heavy.

This room has a door. Maybe I can use it, with my mind. Maybe I can spirit walk into the hallway—but now I see him, at the window, a gargantuan cartoon duck holding a glass of lemonade. "Hey," he says. "Got any grapes?"

IN THIS VERY BIRTH ROOM at the Grace Hospital, I've cut cords after dads have collapsed, syncopal, before they can complete the deed. I've broken the bed, lifting women's legs up in McRoberts position to help free the baby's head in cases of shoulder dystocia. I've helped wheel women from this room to the surgical suite where they hope the obstetrician will cut very, very quickly. Unlike then, I now have the leisure to lounge. The lay person might think catching a baby is a special experience, but the true miracle is having one.

Against the wall directly across from the bed, a large television set is inlaid in a discreet cabinet. Women can watch as they wait for contractions to intensify, at which point their attention turns decidedly inward. Windows look out on the perpetually full parking lot, offering a brooder like me lots of surface area to tether my thought. I'm twenty-four years old, almost done medical school. I feel like I've dared to be here, that *we've* dared to be here. But daring is one thing, doing another.

Court and paternity-reveal talk shows alternate until the evening newscast comes on. Light slowly recedes as the sun descends, my thought a kind of anti-photosynthesis, blooming as the darkness consolidates. As ATV anchor Steve Murphy's potato-head slowly bobs with the unseen teleprompter, Janet's pain begins to crest as serial immensity, receding only slowly and never quite going away, preserving tension. There always is a tide. We watch Steve as biology rises; Steve watches invisible words flowing above our head and speaks them aloud, to us.

"Do you want some beach sounds to play instead?" our labour and delivery nurse asks. Janet shakes her head no. The pain's becoming her entire focus. For her, noise is noxious. For me, it's alterations in brightness.

Closer and closer the pain comes until there is just enough time for her to get breath back; correspondingly, closer and closer the child comes, farther and farther down the vaginal canal, until, finally, the head presents.

Outside, it's completely dark. The television has long been turned off. *American Idol* finally did it—the off-key auditions were too much for Janet, she who has gradually scaled a mountain of pain for an entire day. Soon, time to make the summit. This is all proceeding well. Predictably.

The windows occasionally gleam as headlights from the lot make just the right angle.

She screams at the crowning—the mountain peak—but once the baby's head comes out, she's already on the down slope. The doctor deftly suctions the nose and mouth as the face emerges. I see shoulders, then body. A girl. A Zee.

The scissors pass to me. The taut cord resists the first snip, requiring a second pass.

No one in our family has told us that we made the right decision. Five months into gestation, one in-law said, "You know, they have a thing called abortion. You could have done that. I mean, you're a doctor. It's something you know, right?" Even my mother, devout Catholic, tarried here, imperfect in the faith. Since no one else will tell me what I need to hear, except for BCJ of course, in the birthing room I tell it to myself: *You did the right thing.*

MY BODY AND MIND INCREASE MOMENTUM despite the fact that the drugs are at maximal dose. I am unable to stand still, impervious to sleep, BCJ double-timing my superspeed, completing two laps to my one, twenty to my ten, fist bumping me each time I'm lapped, BCJ no longer at the stripper bar but going full Tony Montana, *Say hello to my little friend,* face buried in the coca.

Dr. Black holds a syringe destined to stick in my ass. In a calm voice, he says, "Shane, we are going to give you some medication to help you." My legs are weighted down by a couple of orderlies, arms too. My head is held to the side, making it mildly hard to breathe. "Haloperidol five mg and Lorazepam two mg," Dr. Black orders. By the sound of his voice, the needle has been passed to someone else and it's about to go in.

"But I'm not psychotic!" I bellow. I *am* psychotic. A sampling of my thoughts:

1. my wife wants to stab me with a kitchen knife through the heart (and I deserve it);
2. Dr. Black is a shoemonster who hoards shoes;

3. the college registrar has burned my resident's license to practise medicine;
4. everyone, everywhere, is out to get me; and, most importantly,
5. BCJ! Is! Real!

"I don't need sedation! I just want to die!"

Pressure on my torso from above makes me forego talking for breathing. A slight wetness on my right buttock. A needle breaks the skin and meets muscle. BCJ, decelerating like a fetal heartbeat, comes to rest. Conked out on the mat next to me, he drools from the drugs. But not me. Me, I got so high that I see Jesus.

JANET CALLS MY NAME. The baby is blue, her cry weak. The obstetrics resident and nurse wrap Zee in blankets, rub her, place her on the incubator. Their calm speed suggests to me a mild alacrity—not enough to call for help, not yet.

Babies perk up, almost always. If the natural history of humans were extrapolated from their first minute on earth, then we would not be successful as a species. Collectively, we would sleep in a brief, blue world.

The resident returns to Janet and deals with the placenta, waiting for it to eject itself, carefully inspecting the bloody pulp for completeness and health. A slight sigh from the nurse pulls my attention back to the baby, who has now pinked up and kicks to punctuate her screams of protest. *How dare you. I was comfy in there.* The nurse places her on Janet's breast.

I'm the accessory in the room, as necessary as the switched-off television set, just a new father who broadcast a promise, a calling yet to be realized as a deed.

MY HEAD, HANDS, AND FEET are fastened down by five-point restraints. A bladder catheter dangles between my legs. How many hours have I been out? Every part of my body *burns*, even the eyelids. I beg to be allowed to move my arms and legs, but there is no one to hear. Except for BCJ, who is dressed up like the cop from the Village People, and is boogying down, lip-syncing "YMCA".

Young man.

Too long later, a nurse comes and releases my left arm as a trial to see if I will behave. I wait for her to start writing in the chart—everything here is pens, is permanent unalterable record, mistakes preserved in ink, nothing is perfect—and then slowly move my left arm to my right side, hoping to release the right arm before anyone can stop me. Wisely, they chose to free my non-dominant arm first. When the first buckle finally comes undone, she screams, "HE'S TRYING TO GET OUT OF THE RESTRAINTS! CODE WHITE!"

Young man.

It takes less than a minute for the team to truss me back in full restraints. My brief, furious expenditure of energy converts the earlier deep ache into agony. Hold a heart in your hands, prevent it from expanding into asystole. Hold a Porsche at maximum throttle, in seventh gear, brakes full on. Jesus, vibrating on the cross, spirit about to be sucked out, but lingering there, gripping each cell, refusing to leave the mortal body, holding on for just a second more carnality, a moment more flesh, the implacability of having to leave and not wanting to go, this desire the perfect opposite of mine.

Young man.

More hours pass. My body settles into a revolting whole pain that comes from being unable to move. I am abject, repeating pathetic pleas from earlier. "Please let me out. Please let me out. Let me free. I'll be good. I promise I'll be good."

But they can't let me out. I can't blame them. I could be free by now, but I can't be. Because of what I did. Because I tried to escape.

No need to be unhappy.

Dr. Black sits in a chair at the right side of the bed. My wife has called. She wants to see me. She cares. I care that she cares, I don't want her to see me like this. This is the worst moment of my life. Black asks, "Can you control yourself so your wife can see you outside of the restraints?" Black repeats himself, slowly, so that I understand. It's as if he's the patient version of my father, asking for a sledgehammer with all the time in the world.

"Yes. I understand. I can control myself. I will follow the rules."

They let out my left arm. *Wait.* My right. *Wait.* My head. *Wait.* Then both my legs.

I will behave. I do not want to be shamed in front of Janet. I wait for her.

ELEMENTS OF THE OBSTETRICAL HISTORY ARE QUANTITATIVE, as if knowledge is precise, measurable. Date of last menstrual period, a calculation with a pregnancy wheel to determine length of gestation, blood pressure, symphysis-fundal height, degree of cervical effacement, head position, urine protein amounts, hemoglobin level.

The birth of Zee didn't feel numerical. Instead, it felt like I stepped outside myself to retrieve a key to the future that, somehow, was buried in the past. As if Janet's cresting pain was the past pushing forward and the receding pain was the present, dragging us out with the tide.

The nurse closes in on Zee's face. "Stork bites," she diagnoses, pointing at Zee's nose. Sensing my confusion, she touches her own nose. Then I suddenly see them: Zee has red marks on either side of her nasolabial folds. *Nevus flammeus nuchae.* "The marks go away," I tell my daughter before I give her back to Janet for more feeding. "Don't worry, they go away as you grow." Protecting Zee from the judgement of others is the first fatherly act I perform. I step out into a long hallway, all the adjoining doors closed to protect the privacy of labouring women in pain.

EIGHTH FLOOR NUMEROLOGY:

3 trips to the Therapeutic Quiet room

2 suicide attempts in the first month

increasing doses of sedatives (now at 2 mg clonazepam bid)

continuous 1:1 supervision for the first month

10 hours in 5 points

start of a trial of Olanzapine 5 mg on day 28

I speak to Dr. Black only when he pays courtesy visits during my inter-regnums in TQ. Little psychotherapy happens on the inpatient ward since one is rather too insane for counselling to be of much use. Chats consist of simple messages that contain imperatives. I'm groggy from the injection from an hour before.

"I often see agitated depression in my elderly patients, and for them I use Olanzapine. Maybe this would make a difference for you too? I know you despise the drug category name, that it's an 'antipsychotic', but I really think you should consider trying it.

But I am not psychotic, I think. The drugs are so thick in my blood-stream, I can only say, "Nnnnnnn."

How many times have I written the words, "Patient has poor insight" into the chart? How many times have I had reality-defying conversations in which they plainly did not believe what was true, simply because their world was not the same consensual reality I lived in? Dr. Black has the knack of suggesting something that is actually a command. As he sits there quietly, I begin to wonder. *Dr. Black is so reasonable. Am I psychotic?*

G, my nurse, enters the code to access the TQ room. Some days, she wears fluffy greens with a pink and turquoise tropical bird pattern. Other days, street clothes. Today all the birds regard me quizzically, wondering what bad things I've done.

Like Dr. Black, G is a People Who Care. Sad, somewhat mom-ish, G shows kindness by listening to the pressured, irrelevant things I have to say, like how much better I am, or that I deserve my shoes. By show-ing me that she's willing to listen, she also shows me *how* to listen, that listening is even possible. Lying prone, my head turned to the left, I try to say "G" to G but only gurgling comes out. Her name's impossible to say. My whole head is brackish, my mouth a producer of air bubbles.

G tries to understand, though—a key feature of People Who Care. She leans closer, says "Yes?" as if it were a question.

I try to say "Yes" too, as if she miraculously understands I'm calling her name, but all that comes out is a yes-like sound: "Yuhhhhhhhh."

This is enough for Dr. Black. "Good. We'll start the medication tomor-row, after you've had a chance to sleep."

THE DAY BEFORE I JUMPED FROM THE BALCONY, Zee tried out the red scooter Janet and I bought her as a birthday present. Holding the scooter, Janet spoke the words I should have spoken as she held Zee steady. I watched them through the window on the third floor, self-confined to quarters.

Zee learned to push off with her free leg. Janet followed Zee as she made ever-widening circles under the cloudless sky on this perfect, late fall morning. From my vantage point, I couldn't see if Janet was smiling. Zee sped up, steering away from the parked cars, and eventually settled upon a happy radius.

Hours later, I heard Zee come in, happy with her lesson and begging to go out again. I remained in my bed, trying to pass undetected. When I did get up, I saw that cars had filled in the space she used.

PEOPLE OF GOOD FAITH, WITHOUT PROOF

My two-year-old son Kaz smashes an ambulance into the small tower of Lego blocks I built for him yesterday, since everything else in the house has already been saved. The ambulance has been busy saving imaginary people for over a year, ever since Kaz learned to walk. Small enough for me to palm, with a now-scuffed right cab light and a crack in the windshield, Kaz's ambulance rushes across carpets and bangs into walls, waiting for no man. *ROOOOOOOO* Kaz screams. *ROOOO* as he bashes it again into the tower.

Firetrucks are *firefucks* and polices are *pleases*—but an ambulance is a *bul-lince*, top of the emergency pantheon, King of All Accidents. If I don't cheer on each smash with a clap or a laugh, he grinds the ambulance into my foot, driving it up my leg towards my head. "Way to save people, Kaz!" I say, giving him what he wants. *ROOOOOOOO* down my leg, now careening towards the mantel.

EVEN MID-MORNING, sun behind cloud can create the effect of a penumbra of fire—Burning Crown Jesus, peeking up from behind the veil of the world. Lights flash atop the Guelph-Wellington Paramedics ambulance, making for a cliché: either headed to a sick person or carrying one, someone needs saving in a hurry.

The sinister ambulances are the quiet ones. Why don't they activate their sirens? What is their purpose? Perhaps they are earmarked to attend slow disasters, mere borderline calamities not worthy of siren-anointed urgency.

Or maybe what's happening inside them is so delicate, so intricate, that the paramedics require absolute concentration to save a life. Or worse: maybe the disaster is so sad, the only proper thing is silent transport of the dead.

The wind's strong today, enough to take a child's toque and whip it down the street. The daycare doors mechanically whine outward, straining against the gusts. Strapped to a gurney, Kaz makes an awful sound: SNAAARRRKKKKLLLLK.

If Kaz were alert, he'd be awestruck: a *real* ride in a *real bul-lince* with real *mens*, the *bu-lincemens* he imagines in the act of saving people, *mens* he makes rush left and right in their vehicles. Mens who are invisible, unseen. Kaz imagined their regular heroism each day, choreographing massive rescues and relief, saving everybody in Guelph every single day of his life. But at the moment, his eyes remain wet and open, gazing somewhere beyond the ceiling. Perhaps he sees Jesus, but I am not privileged to know. I have only my own personal one.

I look past the paramedic and consider instead the differential diagnosis of new-onset seizures: blood in my son's brain; an infection in his meninges; an insatiable tumour; the stroke of God. Though I can't tell how fast we're going, I decide that this ambulance isn't fast enough. I want it to go Kaz velocity, appetite for destruction, gasoline for the machine, dreadnought-ramming speed.

Cars slowly grant right of way to the siren. If Kaz were driving, his hand on top of the ambulance, we'd cleave through cars, lifting them up and over like a cowcatcher, like the bifurcation of dirt from a plough in the field. As we make the turn onto Delhi Street, Kaz's cry becomes sharper, filling the ambulance to resonance. He seems to be returning to where his body lives, as if his body is fighting hard to keep hold of his ghost, pulling it back. His ghost doesn't want to come back, it bellows fury—a life's most concentrated essence, the refusal to do anything, anywhere, *no*. This cry is an otherworldly keen, a reckoning from, or with, the beyond. An artificial sound. A lost noise.

As we pull up to the hospital bays, Kaz opens his eyes, looks from the paramedic to me and back. "D- d- d- d-" he stutters, fighting weakly against the belts securing him to the gurney. "Ddddd. D. D-d-d-d."

Dad? Dead? Dere? Though Kaz and I trained and trained for this moment, it's nothing like we expected—we're not the heroes here. We're townsfolk that need saving, mere pedestrians run over by an indifferent, distracted motorist. Kaz looks down at the straps, realizing that he is bound. He strains his arms against them and, thwarted, starts to cry—a thin, conscious, familiar, querulous cry, the one I've heard so often before, one that comes when he's hungry, soiled, or bored, when something is denied. For the first time, I hear this sound with relief. Like anyone else held against their will, like me, he wants to be free.

AS A PHYSICIAN, I start things off with people by inquiring about their history, reconstructing why they have come. According to my training, which was traditional and part of an undeviating line extending from the eighteenth century and likely quite far into the future, I inquire about a constellation of symptoms according to an approach that conceives of the body as a machine. I glean when each symptom started, worsened, improved, and what might have made it better. Has the pain ever come before? I inquire about the use of drink, drugs, and tobacco. I ask if any illnesses happen to cluster in a patient's family. I was taught in medical school that 80% of the time a patient's illness can be properly diagnosed by taking a history alone, but it has to be a *good* history, a *correct* one.

A tall, thin man clad in light blue hospital scrubs and an unbuttoned lab coat approaches. These details plus the stethoscope around his neck suggest that he is a physician. The speed of his step suggests how much the exigencies of time press upon his professional demeanor. How to connect with patients in the most efficient way possible? What is the perfect balance of engagement and extraction? What is the minimum titration of the human?

"Hi Shane. We've met a few times. I'm Daniel."

I remember. Daniel is the husband of Shelley, a colleague from a medical clinic where I work. Daniel is already known to me as a People Who Care, a doctor on the right side of the line drawn by simple decency and pride, the one BCJ dragged my ass over, some days doing the one-man carry like a firefighter seeing a blaze somewhere off in the distance, running to that fire encumbered, somehow not running away, preventing me from fleeing.

My son lies on a gurney in a major trauma room in the Guelph General Hospital. He keeps trying to sit up, but as soon as he reaches an upright position, he topples over. Before Daniel starts taking a history, reciting the litany of questions I know intimately, he simply watches Kaz sit up, fall over, and try to sit again.

In medical school, we're told to really notice each patient so that we can determine if they are sick. Sometimes, the first five seconds of watching can tell a doctor almost everything they need to know. In addition, this process is a good introduction to any patient. It says: *I notice you. I am closely watching you. You have my complete attention. I am a People Who Care.*

Daniel bends down at the side of the gurney. "Mr. Kazuo? I am Dr. Danny. It is nice to meet you." Daniel grabs Kaz's available left hand and shakes it solemnly with his right. "Oooo, you look very very very strong," he says to Kaz. "Are you strong? Let me see here now. Those are … muscles, no way! Those are super big muscles!" Smiling a doctor-patented, genuine I-Am-A-Very-Nice-Doctor-Smile, one designed to coax kids into torture for their own good, Daniel pretends to measure Kaz's bicep with measuring tape usually used on neonates. "Shane, *look* at the size of these pipes! I mean, he's like Bamm-Bamm Rubble! When Kaz shakes your hand, does he throw you around?"

Kaz slurs a laugh. He likes Daniel. "Doc-tor, doc-tor."

With kids, I too adopt the schtick of a performing clown at a birthday party. The goal is to make their time in health care environments less terrifying, oftentimes the best one can do. Maybe needles. Maybe drugs. Maybe blades. Maybe reductions. But also, maybe a human face.

I worry that this excitement might provoke another seizure, but Daniel is undeterred. He looks in Kaz's ears and shines light in his eyes. Strengthless, Kaz cannot resist, but he also doesn't want to, Daniel has won him over. He wants another Daniel muscle measurement. "Tape," Kaz says. "Tape me. Me tape."

Daniel hands Kaz the tape, but it falls out of Kaz's hands onto the floor. Having connected with his patient, and having performed enough of an exam to ensure that Kaz is not critically ill, Daniel turns to me to take the history. He starts with quick closed-ended questions—all business. "Nurses say no fever today. Did Kaz have a fever in the past week?"

"No."

"Has he been sick in any way? A cough?"

"No."

Then he leaves the narrow runway to rise into a wide-open question: "All right then. What happened, tell me the story."

I feel like a medical student again, overwhelmed by the sheer data of a life, unsure of how to organize it when presenting to a staff physician who, seemingly, has done this work over a long career. Having a sick child has undone all the medicine I thought I knew.

THE PERPETUAL SHADOW SIDE to my conversations with strangers is my non-neurotypicality. In unfamiliar situations, I stiffen, offering less body language. My speech becomes circumlocutory and arcane. When asked a question, I ponder its nature rather than answer. My consciousness descends to floor level and surveys feet, noting shoe type and material. Someone with social skills might smile and sail easily through the social world. Such is my romance: George Clooney of *ER*, that tanned silver fox, smiles at people who smile back, the entire normative universe smiling along with them. Clooney, of course, wears impeccable, shining oxfords. But on this off-work day, I take after my main man BCJ: beat-up sandals.

Hospital workers can be differentiated by their clothing. Nurses wear colourful greens; physios, stylish and tight-fitting clothes; occupational therapists adopt blocky, prow-like garb; physicians sport white coats or, if less exposed to blood and guts in the course of daily work, they don sweaters and dress shirts marking them as medical gentry; orderlies and sanitation workers tend to wear basic greens with nothing in their pockets; maintenance workers carry telltale tools. If ever in doubt about the type of worker, look at the shoes. The more expensive the shoes, the likelier it is that the person is a physician or an executive. The more functional the shoe, the higher the chance that the wearer is on their feet all day. Trust in those with the comfortable shoes, go in fear of Manolo Blahnik high heels and Louis Vuitton oxfords. (Run screaming from bowties.)

Kaz wears Superman sneakers with Velcro straps. All around us in the emergency department, a sea of white sneakers swirls around an occasional riotously coloured pair of Crocs. Safe, safe for now, from a leather interloper, from a sharky pump.

KAZ'S NECK UNNATURALLY EXTENDS ON MY KNEE. People walk up and down the hall in front of our bay—professionals following the shoe code, but also dishevelled and scared family members in street clothes, fellow travellers living out our worst fears as we witness family members suffer. The general public today tends to prefer sneaker, with the occasional pair of basic block shoes. Everywhere I look in the bays, I see family members falling somewhere on a spectrum of distress. Everywhere on our side of the line, People Who Care. Raising autism radar from floor-level, I feel, before I see, that the emergency department has no windows.

"Frrrrnk," Kaz says. "Frrrnk frrrnk frrnk frrrnk frrrnk," a slurred enunciation of 'drink.'

As opposed to regarding the variety of shoe species, everyone stares into a monoculture of cellphone: nurses, doctors, paramedics, patients, family members. When I trained as a doctor, no one could use cellphones in the emergency department, the fear being that cardiac equipment might malfunction due to spectral interference. Now the fear is different and exists on our side of the line, that phones distract staff too much. For we need your complete attention, our loved ones require devotion.

Emergency departments don't have windows for reasons to do with light and location. I know this, but knowledge doesn't change the fact that I need a window. I call Janet at the Microscope Room, a place where she examines the cells of dead animals to determine cause of death. Tara, her pathology colleague, answers the phone. "No, she's not here right now, Shane—I'll leave a note for her at her desk."

Perhaps a different outlet. I send my wife a text instead. *Kaz had a seizure. We are at GGH emergency. He's on my lap, not moving much. He's stopped crying though, I think that's good. He's watching everybody. He wants D-R-I-N-K but that's not allowed until the doctor says so.*

A sudden vision of Janet materializing: Kaz says, "MOOOMMMMYY." I hold her as she holds the boy in her arms. I exude George Clooney-ness, smiling as if my facial muscles exist in harmony with the world, a perfectly white and calibrated smile that revolves around the axis of my oxford shoes, head spinning exorcist-style.

"Is he going to die?" Janet asks.

In my imagination, Clooney loses his smile, his handsome face now blank as mine, reduced to living on our side of the line, sitting next to a sick loved one. He's in bare feet, his soles and toes cracked at their foundation, dyshidrotic, no green room moisturizer available for miles.

"I don't think so. He's conscious. Thirsty. The doctor needs to figure out what happened."

Kaz remains slack, his body still requiring support. Drool drips out of the left side of his chin. He alternates grunts with slurred takes on the word 'drink.'

"Do you think I should come now?"

Aren't you here, with us, already?

"Frrnk."

Clooney looks up, startled by the sudden appearance of Amal, his wife. She wears her husband's forgotten smile and shares his former extravagant taste in shoes—in this case, elegant Antonio Vietri Moon Stars. Her hands rub his blank face, trying to get the motor going. Nothing doing, warming up his million-dollar mug won't resuscitate the *orbicularis orus*, aka smile muscle. Thankfully, she has packed a hospital bag, and she pulls out a set of Aubercy diamond-studdeds.

Daddy likes. Wattage returns. Clooney smiles again, the couple now a perfect match. His and Hers smiles, perfected over long repetition, a hundred thousand red carpets and exponents of cameras.

"Just a second," I say, putting the phone down. A nurse asks me to hold Kaz so she can draw blood. Another nurse comes, then another. We're surrounded. I lay Kaz down on the bed. One nurse takes his legs, the other his right arm and head, the other pins his left arm to draw the blood. Kaz doesn't resist, the nurses talking to him as if they love him, telling him he is a good boy, so good. They are smiling, smiling, smiling, cooing, smiling. So good, the best one we've had in so long, wow, good job here dad, this boy is super.

My father, repeating *You are bad, bad, so bad …*

"Frrrnk", Kaz begs. "Frrnk."

Is this a heavenly host of angels, a swarm of People Who Care? The needle punctures the vessel wall and tubes of every colour fill with miraculous blood. "Shane?" Janet asks, her voice breaking on the phone. Minutes have ticked by with the phone pressed to my ear, no idea how it got there. I set it down, didn't I?

An old woman on a wheelchair rolls down the hall, IV pole maneuvered by her daughter. The mother has a left leg twice as large as her right one. A bag with the word 'cefazolin' hand-printed on pink tape drips clear liquid into her arm.

As usual, I play the diagnosis game. I'm always playing, silently assessing people in line at a movie theatre, at restaurants, sitting on streetcars or in the clinic. Type 2 diabetes complicated by cellulitis? Is amputation necessary, not acutely, but in a few days' time? Is the daughter taking her mother out to smoke?

When a doctor observes details, medical narratives naturally spring to mind. Doctors see and hear the hidden things in their offices, but doctors also see hidden things in plain sight.

"Yes, come now," I say to my wife.

KAZ'S DROOL SOAKS THROUGH MY SHIRT, pooling in the umbilicus. The ceiling of the Guelph General Hospital is alabaster white. Somewhere, a voice is speaking. Not from the ceiling. From in front of me.

"So, let me repeat what you told me so I can be sure I have it correct. Kaz fell, and he seemed to shake. As far as you know, something might have happened in the car, and he fell and was unresponsive for a time at the daycare."

When I was twelve years old, I got up from my one-piece wooden desk during social studies, requiring the diagonal metal support bar to stand. I remember wanting to tell Mrs. Clark, my teacher, that I was going to die. Telling her seemed conscientious, I thought she should be informed. So that she could plan, ensure that the pencil counts were right at the end of the day. I wasn't in pain, I was in absence, the world slipping away, the ceiling, or something beyond the ceiling, pulling me, infusing warmth.

Before I could reach her the room went away from me. I felt as if I were shrinking, and the tables and chairs and children around me growing—what I recognize now as a case of Alice in Wonderland Syndrome, a well-documented seizure phenomenon. The room's colours washed out to a solid white. Laughter roared down from the ceiling—a man's mocking voice, but no man I knew.

Silly Shane.

Silly Shane.

I collapsed. A few minutes later, I returned to consciousness and the room resumed its usual colours and dimensions. No ambulance was called, and I saw no doctor. Instead, Mrs. Clark returned to the front of the classroom to resume reading from Ray Bradbury's *The Martian Chronicles:*

> "It may be, sir, that we're looking upon a phenomenon that, for the first time, would absolutely prove the existence of God, sir."
>
> "There are many people who are of good faith without such proof, Mr. Hinkston."

Daniel says, "This could be a seizure disorder but it's hard to say. Maybe Kaz had a fever that went down before we measured it. Febrile seizures would be the best thing. We'll do blood work and observe him. I'll come back and finish the rest of my exam when he's more active."

A set of elevator shoes scuds by—a chopper patrolling the delta. Recognizing that Kaz is asleep, the human in the shoes hovers, quietly pulling two small packages of Oreo cookies out of their green work vest. Elevator shoes sets them on a ledge near the sliding doors, taking pains not to crinkle the packaging, and then scuds away.

When I walked home from school the day of my first seizure, stumbling in a different register of light, I heard more laughter, but this time it emanated from the snow itself, echoing everywhere. I probably had another partial seizure and didn't know. Maybe a series of them. The snow was whiter than I thought it could ever be—an impossible, glowing white. The newly over-imbued world took a few more days to lose its additional radiance.

Twenty-five years later, Mrs. Clark's reading voice returns to me in the Guelph General as I look at my son. It's as if she's in the ceiling, on the other side of the mineral fibre panels: "On nights when the wind comes over the dead sea bottoms and through the hexagonal graveyard, over four old crosses and one new one, there is a light burning in the low stone hut, and in that hut, as the wind roars by and the dust whirls and the cold stars burn...."

The cold stars, the burning crown, sky as stained-glass planetarium, the glittering floor a pocket dimension of different-coloured suns, Aldebaran, Antares, Arcturus, Betelgeuse, Spica, red, gold, yellow, green, white, Rigel as Orion's blue suede shoe, actual shoes—a pair of dusty sandals peeks underneath the closed curtain, pedicured toes rippling up and down.

AN ANNOUNCER INTONES, *"Enter Burning Crown Jesus* is proud to deliver you an episode on delusions. Fixed false beliefs. Full fathom five. Christ—is he with us, or not with us? Is he against us? Is this Christ, the one wearing the burning crown, the one producing this program— is he a delusion? We take you to an unethical experiment run by a little boy—who has very naughtily NOT sought Institutional Review Board approval—on his doddering grandpa."

A little boy's voice asks, "What is a delusion?"

A German-accented voice answers. "A delusion is an unusual belief that resists counterevidence and is not given up easily in the face of challenge."

The little boy says, "I am pushing a button, you are receiving a thousand volts of electricity, please answer the question better next time. SNAAARRRKKKKLLLLK. What is a delusion?"

A German-accented voice answers, "An act of imagination!"

The little boy voice says, "Correct. Remember to use Silly Shane in your answers. Why do people develop delusions?"

The German voice says, "One of the more compassionate hypotheses as to why people experience delusions is that, when confronted with new experiences, they overvalue the power of the new experience and undervalue the stabilizing weight of previous experience. When in a new situation, such people are completely in the moment, given over to the new, and they are open to a range of new possible explanations for the current experience. Take, for example, Shane. Shane is in the hospital, with his son. This is a horrible new experience. But in the mirror, he catches a reflection, a strange shape, an odd glimmer. And he explains this new experience, this strangeness, not as many others would, they being stabilized by the ballast of previous experience. Others might say, 'That's a window. Light hits it and makes reflections.' But Silly Shane thinks he sees Jesus. Maybe there's a reason he thinks Jesus specifically— perhaps childhood experiences, perhaps cultural ubiquity of that religious symbol. But as compared to someone who is not psychotic, Shane's perceptual experiences point to Jesus as an ultimately integrated possibility and credible explanation for the phenomenon.

"Further—I trust my answers may be full?—delusions are often the product of previous hallucinations. This creates a chicken-or-egg paradox, but the idea is: hallucinate Jesus. Then believe Jesus is real, naturally enough! Then believe that your entire life is a conversation with this reality, that your existence is informed by conversations with a deity. The hallucinations and delusions kindle one another until it is difficult to separate which is which. Is this radio program, for example, an auditory hallucination, an instance of, as they say, 'hearing voices'? Or does it exist instead as a fully integrated reality involving tactile, visual, and other auditory phenomenon? Or is the nature of our reality itself impoverished, in the sense that data is only a fraction of the creation of consciousness, with the bulk of the experience generated by the mind—what might be, according to another way of thinking, a purely delusory phenomenon, one involving reasoning and cognition rather than sensory data? It is not for me to say, though I do think it strange that the philosophers privilege the sense organs so highly in their formulations. Belief in the world comes from within."

The little boy voice says, "We accept this answer, though much more *could* be said. Next question. If Burning Crown Jesus were a delusion, then what kind of delusion is he?"

The German voice answers, "BCJ is a monothematic delusion. These kinds of delusions tend to cohere around a single theme, whereas poly-thematic delusions involve a range of both related and unrelated delusions that create a larger matrix of bizarre belief. For Silly Shane, who is the subject here, the protagonist who may or may not be experiencing delu-sions—Shane seems to suffer (if he is suffering, for he would not deem it so) the monothematic kind. If Shane were asked why his brand of crazy were monogamous rather than polygamous, he would respond with an answer based in the delusion itself, which is what all the delusory do. He would insist 'BCJ is real' and try to convince you of the fact. I hope, however, that by connecting his profound belief in the reality of BCJ with the irony of the monothematic delusion, he may be able to make some progress. Shane may respond positively to the insight that his monothematic delusion is for a monotheistic faith. He may perceive a symmetry here, and in making that connection, we hope we can create a small bit of separation between Shane and his tightly held conviction about the reality of BCJ.

The little boy asks, "But what would he do, once BCJ were success-fully exorcised from his life?"

The German voice answers, "His delusory capacity may simply create monothematic content of a different sort. Or, he may prove profoundly lonely without his imaginary friend. Or, he may die without this protective delusion in place, thereby solving the existential problem of loneliness— a condition that has plagued him for his entire life, one that, in another irony, likely suggested Jesus as an ideal companion, someone who would literally die to save Shane."

And now a word from our sponsors. Here at Big Christianity, we ...

ONCE UPON A TIME, A MONSTER

Once upon a time, a boy was born in rural New Brunswick during the Second World War. He became a binge drinker and was often violent—especially towards the women in his life, including my mother, his second wife. I was his firstborn son, too slow and strange to understand his commands or develop strategies to mitigate his abuse.

My father, considered by many as a bad man, was, in fact, neurodivergent himself. He was taken to psychiatrists when he was quite young, but no help could be given to control his behaviour, no diagnosis to adequately brand him. The sketch provided by others of my father as a child is hazy and indistinct, but it always has the same taint. If he did something unspeakably transgressive, I was never told. The only thing I know is he was somehow 'bad.' Vaguely bad. Generally bad.

On the first floor of St. Michael's Hospital in Toronto in the year 1999, I find my father in a dank, delirium-inducing chamber. He fell from the top of his semi-truck the day before. Horrid clear goop pools in the medial canthi of his eyes. The staff shaved his face—it's smoother than usual. The endotracheal tube snaking from his mouth gathers moisture in its curvature. Condensation clouds the interior; in one section, water moves back and forth, a tide.

If the gods sleep, do they sleep like this, connected to the neon gases of a narcotized universe? My thoughts attach to the tube, to its sections of clearness and clarity. He's not dead yet, but I'm not relieved by the fact. I'm neutral, the dead core of being currently unthreatened and yet not safe, never safe, the past eating the ground I stand on. I sit on a hard plastic chair next to the bedside. With no window in this place for my thoughts to flow back and forth, my mind extends back into the past.

ONCE UPON A TIME, there was a garage that contained numerous tools that a little boy didn't know how to use. The boy thought they all looked similar and did many of the same things. Hedge shears. Vise. Pliers. Saw. Axe. Hammer. Screwdrivers of a thousand colours and lengths. A sledgehammer.

"Boy, go and get the sledgehammer," said a man who stood in a small, harrowed field, his profile against the sun.

The boy was in his own world. Thoughts extended out of the boy, a riot of ideas. They flowed away from the man because he was scary. They hid from the man. Whenever there was a window, the boy's thoughts drifted there. Without a window, they often shot straight up to the sun.

"BOY. GIT ME THE SLEDGEHAMMER!" the man shouted, and somehow the boy was running before he even understood what he was doing or was supposed to do. He ran in the direction of the garage, and, miraculously, the image of the sledgehammer was in his mind. It had a chipped end. The metal part was blue. The handle was long, smooth, and grainy. Tightly holding his one thought—the image of the sledge— the boy walks in.

His legs had brought him into the garage, about a hundred feet from the other side of the house. The boy's thoughts began to multiply and take on different forms. His legs, having stopped, no longer expended anxious energy stemming from the existential fear that he would die—a fear given him by the man. The boy knew there was only one person who would kill him. He had always known this. He thinks: *where is the sledge where is the sledge where is the sledge?*

The thought becomes a horde of mental locusts, a suffocating confetti, a flight of arrows. The boy runs from either side of the garage and back, stepping and re-stepping in its stains, noting, again and again, the hammers, screwdrivers, pliers, and clippers. But not the sledge.

A full five minutes goes by until the boy hears, "WHAT THE FUCK ARE YOU DOING? I NEED THE FUCKING SLEDGEHAMMER!"

The boy stops. His thoughts stop. He has no capacity now except, in the last few seconds he will be alive, to regard the man before the blow comes. The boy looks up. The man blocks out the rest of the street. He looms huge and high. His right arm extends out. The boy watches the arm with fascination and hears some sound in his body—a rhythmic thrum.

The man picks up the sledgehammer that was always in plain view, that was easy to see, that had been waiting all along like a moral, a reckoning. And he goes into the backyard with it. The boy is left alone. He's not dead.

Somehow this memory is about how the boy tried so hard and couldn't, about how the man was scary, but also about how the boy has to decide what to do next—to sprout wings and fly into the sun, or drink down cans of motor oil, or load the shotgun mounted above the work desk and put it in his mouth, or to go again into the backyard and help the man with his work.

The boy runs into the backyard. The man he has become, me, returns to my father's bedside at St. Michael's Hospital in the year of our Lord 1999. The old man's mechanical breathing strikes me as analogous to the repetition of trauma.

ONCE UPON A TIME, the ICU bed closest to my father's was occupied by an old man who suffered a massive stroke. His frail Italian wife sits next to him daily, just like I do with my father. She and I are the designated watchers. As I leave my post one evening, she follows after, croaking, "You're a good boy, a good son. You sit next to your father every day. I have three boys. They won't come here. When I tell them about their father, they yell, they hang up on me. They call their father 'bastard.'"

"Mine's a bastard, too," I say, slowly shaking my head in simple awe. To consider my father's life is to be amazed. How did he not die? And why didn't I? "But someone has to be there in case they wake up, right?" For I am a People Who Care, either a tricked or true believer to whom love is duty.

Outside the ICU, several wall-mounted angel statues gaze, part of an iconography straight from my childhood's central casting department. A series of plaques tell the story of St. Michael's Hospital when it was run by the Catholic church. Green tapestries feature saints with burning hearts and glowing haloes. Just like the stained-glass windows of my youth, the foyer walls declare that extravagant beauty is the healing you need.

A group of nuns wearing pristine habits eat lunch in the overpriced cafeteria. All are elderly except for one young woman who holds the attention of her seniors. She's a fine bride of Christ, her attractive shape unobscured by the black fabric. Assuming the eldest is the authority, I interrupt their conversation and ask the most senior-appearing nun a question. "Who was St. Michael?" The nuns look at one another as if to decide, collectively, if they should speak to the infidel. "It's okay, I'm Catholic," I add. "Or I used to be. Anyway, I'm confirmed. I just can't remember who St. Michael is."

I suspect, looking back now, that I was profoundly unwell. Perhaps their hesitation had nothing to do with presumed lack of faith and everything to do with my shabby comportment. But sisters, it is written in Matthew 25: *Inasmuch as ye have done it unto one of the least of these my brethren, ye have done it unto me.*

"St. Michael is also known as Michael the Archangel, the angel who leads God's armies in the war in heaven," the young nun says with a shrug. "That's an easy one. Have you been to church lately?"

"No, I haven't," I say, retreating to the ICU, where I sit in a hard chair at the right hand of my father.

ONCE UPON A TIME, Burning Crown Jesus was intubated. He neither died, was buried, or rose again—he merely lay comatose, insensate, requiring rotisserie by nurses so that he wouldn't develop bed sores on his godly body. Once upon a time, Burning Crown Jesus swung a sledgehammer as high as he could into the sky, seeking deliverance. Jesus tracked the sledge as if he were fielding a fly ball and, because he could have been the most talented outfielder who ever lived, Burning Crown Jesus placed his head at the impact point of the sledge and waited, knowing it would come. Bliss. Bless. Once upon a time, Burning Crown Jesus looked at his mortal family through the glass—they were inside the house, restful —and jumped from a height. Once upon a time, Burning Crown Jesus ingested enough medication to slay a city, the pasted overflow running down his chin. Once upon a time, there was a thing called trauma and the character called Silly Shane kept walking through it as if it were a hallway or road, kicked out at different points on the timeline, all of them traumatic, all of them involving the death of Christ, all of them seeming like a nightmare, some of them involving his actual father, some of them involving his own actual history. But remember: each time Christ dies, Shane is saved. Even the comatose god, the one being kept alive by artificial means—another prolonged, intractable save. For every so often, there needs to be a place for this nonlinear Shane to go that can hold him when he is dead to the world, but yet not dead. Every so often again, Shane is actually the one intubated, turned by the nurses. Every so often, the love story itself keeps him alive, and BCJ recedes into the background, given a chance to rest up and be ready for the next intercession.

ONCE UPON
A NAME

Why is it that complications *always seem so tidy in retro-spect? Something happens, which leads to something else happening, and so on, until the present arrives and there's nothing left to explain, only circum-stances. When looked at backwards, malpractice is a form of prophecy. Why is it that we never expect trouble until trouble occurs, and from that point on, complications are expected? Why do we invest meaning in events when they might be random? Why reach for fate or faith as explanations? What is the point of imperfect miracles? Let us ask Burning Crown Jesus these, and other questions, later on* Enter Burning Crown Jesus. *But first, a word from our sponsor...*

"MOMMY. MOMMY SOON. Mommy soon. Me Mommy soon." Kaz com-forts himself by kicking his legs rhythmically against my shins. Drool continues to pour out of his mouth.

Daniel returns, rocking slightly on his tiptoes, workload threatening to literally tip him over. "Well, Shane, the good news is Kazuo's blood work is normal. No white count, electrolytes fine." Daniel bends down to eye-level with Kaz. "So how are you now, Kazuo?"

"Not. Sick. Any. More!" Kaz yells each word.

"Good! You look like the healthiest boy ever to me. But I need to check out your muscles to make sure, okay? I'm the doctor. I check muscles." In a gesture that must endear Daniel to most of the parents and children he encounters, he raises his right arm and flexes. His head turns slowly to look at the modest muscle straining past the green shirt. "See? Just like this. I'm Muscle Doctor. But you, you're ... Musclemans!"

Kaz is won over. Daniel is entertainment. Daniel is cool. Kaz raises his right arm to try to mimic Daniel, but he just holds his arm out straight, then covers his eyes.

Daniel performs an age-appropriate neurological exam on my son, keeping it fun the whole way through. "Do you hear the funny sounds in the hall, Kaz? That's *beeping*, Kaz. That's *alarms*. Do you see the wheel-chair people? Oh you do? I check their muscles too. All I do all day is muscles. Your muscles, their muscles. You're Musclemans, Kaz. Your name is Musclemans."

Kaz likes this new name. "Smans. Me smans smans smans."

Daniel turns to me and says, "No focal findings. Power is good, reflexes fine."

"But he's ataxic, he falls after just a step," I say.

"Yeah, that's what happens, right? Kids lose their balance after seizures. He just looks too good right now, too bright, for this to be meningitis. I'm consulting Peds, they'll talk to you about what to do next. Things are good right now, Shane. It might not have even been a seizure, you know?"

If not a seizure, then what do we call it? The Kaz-Almost-Dieds? Daniel sees the package in the sink. "Musclemans, you like cookies? Build some muscle on *cookies*!"

Kaz loves Daniel. "Yes. Candy. Smans smans smans."

"Okay, Musclemans. Dad of Musclemans, these are the doctor's orders: give Musclemans cookies." Daniel raises his arm, as if to salute, but instead he flexes his bicep again. He walks out into the hall holding that posture and disappears from sight.

"Candy!" Kaz demands. "Not. Sick. Any. More!"

I take the Oreos from the sink and give Kaz one of two. "That one! That one!" he yells, meaning he wants both. One wafer in the church, two cookies in the emergency department. He rubs them around his mouth, the external shells blackening his lips and cheeks.

Janet appears at the doorway, pausing there. She wears medical paja-mas, sky-blue ones from Ontario Veterinary College, her hair pulled into a tight bun so no strands drag in corpses from the post-mortem lab. Her happy face unsettles me until I realize she's coming at this the opposite way, to a son who's moving and responsive, in the hands of a parent, *alive*. Not a son heading to an ambulance, one held between worlds by an implacable force, but one who has survived the inciting drama. A son with Cookie Face.

"Mommy!" Kaz screams in complete jubilation, sliding off my lap with soggy cookie mush in each hand. After three steps, he falls, mush plopping on the floor. Janet picks Kaz up and lets him nuzzle her neck, crumbs wetly transferring.

Kaz looks down for his cookies. "Candy, candy, candy!"

"What's happening?" she asks.

I say, "We're waiting for a consult. Tests so far are normal."

Kaz thinks she's talking to him. He says, "I smans."

While he's distracted, I move to stand on the mush. He squirms out of Janet's grasp, takes a step towards the bed—and falls to the floor. Since walking won't work, he crawls around looking for traces of Oreo.

Janet walks to where I sit and presses my head against her chest. Her neck is wet, with sparkling black dust. "You must have been terrified," she says.

I have no idea of time after she says this.

I NEED A NAME. Janet named our firstborn, making it my responsibility to name our second child. My privilege. If the child's female, the job is already done—we'll name her Sonnet after the most beautiful poetic form in English, a form as intricate as a poet might wish. For over fifteen years, I've wished fourteen-lined regular word-shapes into perfection. Failing each time—but perfection is original sin, the idea that what we are, what we do, isn't good enough.

Like the sonnet, human beings rhyme and have spirit. The opening octave is a version of a life before the volta, or turn, lines that define us before we are changed. The closing sestet upends the naïve life, lifting it closer to understanding. The terminal couplet sears the realization, brands it molten upon our backs. Every human out there has a rhyming couplet in their heart capable of defining their existence. Mine is:

And some may never, a great poet wrote.
Feel flames from the crown char your throat.

Maudlin, but at least I know how I'm branded.

I need a name for a boy too, though, and sonnet-writing hasn't helped. Perhaps the coming child is *vers libre,* resistant to stricture and structure? I try out a variety of names in poems that have no strict form, poems that—independent of my plan or intention—won't conform to rhyme scheme, meter, or larger organizational structure. Chaotic things that, though they reflect the human spirit, don't embody the larger human sense, meaning the symmetry and inevitability of our mortal bodies. Biblical names like:

Abaddon
Abdiel
Boaz
Ebenezer
Japheth
Nicodemus
Zebulon
Zipporah

The bible loves Z names. The baby name book offers more normie suggestions:

Ethan
Aiden
Lucas
Kaden
Jayden
Nathan
Logan
Noah

Vowel-rich, almost all either suggesting "and" or "end" at their terminus, no name stands out. Amongst the choices, my personal inclinations slightly incline toward the "end" names, but my parental hope prefers the ampersand. Even so, none of the names come alive in poems that aren't themselves alive.

One night, BCJ appears, and says, "I appreciate you going old skool, but maybe you could just pick your favourite poet? I mean, other than me, of course."

Has the rain a father? Or who has begotten the drops of dew? A vision comes to me of a stand of pines and birches leaning back from an old logging road.

Alden Nowlan, created in mine own image. A Maritime poet like me. Like me, his father was an alcoholic. Like me, Nowlan was non-neurotypical. I once read his books during class in medical school, his poems teaching me the opposite of what bullies do: that emotion is everything in this life, that it's okay to display. In one poem, a mysterious naked man takes to the sky as a subversion of toxic masculinity; in another, a drunk man listening to folk music connects with intellectually disabled children that he recognizes are connected to him somehow (and probably more profoundly than he knew); and in one more, the poet reflects on how he alone knows how empty his house stands without the presence of Claudine, his wife. In almost every poem, the creating consciousness is profoundly self-aware, an awareness born of being *made* self-aware. Nowlan was bullied into realizing the human condition, and the poems are a testament to a world he built himself: one where love could be found.

I know no living Aldens, though; indeed, I've never met one. "Alden" is a name from another age, deriving from the 'Ealdwine' of Old English that means 'old friend.' No one else likes the Alden idea—not my wife, patients, colleagues, or old friends.

Names contain fateful information. They inform destiny, are akin to diagnoses. Names have to be right. On July 21, 2008, the day before Janet's scheduled induction, I ask Janet, "Maybe Alden can be the boy's middle name?"

Hovering over a suitcase containing a veterinary textbook, a bottle of apple juice, and a new maternity dress, Janet looked up at me. "Okay," she says. "But what about a first name?"

FROM UNDER THE BED, Smans' voice demands, "More."

I push closer to Janet, put my hand on her abdomen. Something foolish comes out of my mouth. "They're not supposed to get sick, right?"

Funny fact about any graveyard in Canada of a significant size: they contain whole regiments of battered stones that extend for hundreds of feet, bearing the names of infants who died during the first influenza pandemic, the span of date of birth to date of death truncated to just the base year, 1918, all of these stones bearing the same accursed inscription: *Suffer the little children to come unto me, and forbid them not.*

Not cool, BCJ. I make a mental note to have him buy the next round at Land O.

Her hand moves to my hair. She bends down to see Kaz under the bed. "Under-the-bed monster! Under-the-bed-monster!" she gasps in mock alarm, playing the game Kaz needs. From where he is, he can see all the feet and lower legs moving back and forth across the department, just no torsos or heads. We have the same focus.

The game is not enough. Food is more powerful. "More!"

What is this place of feet and cookies, of name bands and tests that are normal? The Guelph General Hospital feels less like a place of healing and more like an alternative church that houses human frailties according to biomedical faith. The sick wait to learn if they will be saved or sacrificed. The verdict of thumbs up or down from the emperor must wait. Most of the time, the emperor's thumb extends sideways, suspended in between.

Janet smiles at the monster under the bed. The monster flexes its muscles. "I smans mons-ter," a voice declares proudly.

She reaches under the bed to poke the belly of smans. "Cookie muscle," she teases.

"More!" he demands.

Beyond the threshold of the room, Daniel hurries down the hall, arms swinging at his sides, his dark blue Crocs squeaking on the floor. Perhaps he just stepped in blood.

I'M SEATED BY A LARGE WINDOW, searching the universe for a name. I wish it were out there, but the only thing I could hope to find in the glass is Burning Crown Jesus, and he doesn't make suggestions. He only listens.

Janet's fully dilated. We wait for Dr. Wine, the obstetrician, to say it's okay to push. He's short, hirsute, and seems irritated with the nurses as a default. Beyond our quite large birthing room, I see him flit past the doorframe on this big day for babies in the city of Guelph. The dry-erase board is full of female names who will soon be acquainted with their miracles.

Perhaps the baby will be a girl, Sonnet her form.

Janet's pushing. The doctor must have said it was okay. Somehow, he arrived. On Janet's belly are electrodes that sense the strength of uterine contraction. The doctor already affixed an internal monitor to the baby's head some time ago. Two curves undulate on a monochrome screen: big mountains denoting contraction and relaxation, and a slowly oscillating curve reflecting the baby's heart rate decelerating with the clench, and then speeding up with release.

From my time spent on obstetrics rotations, I recall the kinds of problems that result in fetal distress. Worse, I also remember how the whole departmental system is predicated on only one disaster happening at a time. What if two women were simultaneously having complications? What if the obstetrician were in the operating room doing a C-section, or frantically flailing in an open abdomen to staunch a possibly fatal postpartum hemorrhage, while a woman over on the birthing unit needed urgent forceps or else fetal demise? It seems unreasonable to expect disasters in series when everyone knows that they happen in parallel, everything going to hell all at once, like back in 1918.

Name name name I need a name name name.

I've never attended a delivery when there wasn't a name ready to meet the child, though there have been many children not yet ready to meet the name, that would never have the breath to hear the name.

The key to being a doctor is to be calm. When it comes to obstetricians, this is doubly true. For in every birthing room, a baby might die, or a mother might die. I am not a calm doctor. I work in an office all day, pretending that the disasters are distant, headed hospitalward. I prefer disasters to be far away or heading there.

Janet periodically crushes my hand, the baby's heart rate increasing and decreasing in concert with her grip. Dr. Wine dons his gloves, gown, and rubber boots, his professional forecast always calling for blood. In his garb, he resembles a firefighter, and he behaves like one, dousing red blazes in each room. There are so many ways a possible fire can burn out of control, so many places it can go.

IN THE GOSPEL OF JOHN, there is perhaps the most famous phrase in all of the bible: "Jesus wept." Perhaps a function of that fame is the phrase's poetic economy. As the story goes, Jesus learns of his friend Lazarus's death, and, upon later meeting Lazarus's distraught sisters Martha and Mary, Jesus breaks down crying, overcome by their grief. I find the tears in this instance profoundly moving and not at all ironic, as per the contemporary usage, because of where it appears in its sequence. Earlier, Christ practically boasts to Martha that he is "the resurrection, and the life: he that believeth in me, though he were dead, yet shall he live: and whosoever liveth and believeth in me shall never die." As if to say: no biggie, sis, Jesus has got you, my best bro will be up in no time. He even challenges her with a question, to check whether she actually believes. But when he gets a double dose of grief upon meeting the second sister, Mary, his confidence cracks, the bravado flags. Seeing her, Christ cannot shake how profound an end death is, that it robs the living of their love. Even though my entire delusory matrix depends on the wholesale belief that Christ is lord and savior with the power of everlasting life—his superpowers get top billing, out of self-interest—I am most moved not by Jesus's death, his conscious sacrifice, nor even his infamous moment of doubt on the cross, but by his grief for a dead man he loved. Rather than engage in a delusory version of the passion in which I try to comprehend Christ's agony on the cross, I just sit on a ward and cry, communing with how low and broken we are by the sickness of our loved ones.

KAZ THROWS A COOKIE AT JANET to punctuate his demands. "Mommy!" One word to convey volumes: Mommy I don't like this, Mommy you are the proxy of my discontent, Mommy I am bored. Mommy mommy

mommy. *Mommy:* the omniprotest of children. But Kaz, your mother listens carefully. Being the normal parent, she carefully follows instructions and must be the one to convey information to others. My job is just to feel, to know when something's not right. Being unbalanced, I'm closer to unbalancing as a process. Possessing an inner impurity or difference, I am positioned to sense when all is not well. I feel deep inside when things aren't right.

Things aren't right. Discharged, we walk out of the building into the mid-afternoon sun, the hospital's fluorescent lighting no competition for the sky's wattage. Looking down at the snow is no reprieve, for it radiates more intensely than the milder blue above; even Janet's eyes reflect the glare. I think of Russian holy icons, thaumaturgy creating the iconostasis, how the individual artist is humble in the face of God, is merely God's instrument. Janet and I each hold one of Kaz's hands. He swings between us, his weight pulling my right shoulder down.

THE BABY CROWNS AND HOLDS, but there's nothing about this moment that feels like a pause. In fact, Janet's agonized body is straining to hold back the inevitable. Her sternocleidomastoid muscles are fully unfurled flags. This biology cannot stop, there will be an expulsion, the birth plot must resolve.

"Don't push, Janet, don't push." Dr. Wine's voice seems smaller, gentler when not issuing orders to the nurses. "We need to take this slow. Okay?"

Janet, whose eyes are closed, her face contorted, simply nods through the pain.

"Okay, Janet. Just a little push more. Very little. I know it feels like one big push and it'll all be over, but just a little bit, don't be tempted. Okay. Go."

Like a shaken champagne bottle's cork, the head pops into view. Janet's face flows from agony to a sudden relief, as if a torturer operating the rack increased the pull as a pulse, but then set it back to two lower levels of tension.

No idea to know if this is a boy or a girl—all baby faces are sexless. Visible around the baby's neck is a thin, bluish cord. Dr. Wine does not tell Janet this. Instead, he says, "Still *don't* push, Janet, okay? I just need to suction out the baby's nose and mouth."

Dr. Wine says nothing to our birthing nurse either but they are clearly silently communicating. The nurse already has the small suction bulb in hand. She leans in underneath Dr. Wine, who slightly bends forward as if he were a bridge that lifts to let large ships pass by. Wine's left hand still rests against the baby's head, as if he were holding back the tides. His gloved right index finger extends laterally in line with the cord, and then curls underneath, the maneuver intended to put as little tension on the cord as possible.

I realize I am not breathing. I see something else. There is a knot in the cord. Somehow, I am breathing even less.

Wine's finger lifts. He doesn't tug, but instead just steadily tries to cinch the cord over the head. He makes it as far as the child's ear until the cord snaps. Pulsatile blood spurts out of the placental end, of little consequence because Janet has a large reservoir, but the part continuous with the baby's umbilicus siphons a much more precious reserve. The baby will bleed out if the cord is not clamped, but the baby isn't out yet, there's nothing to clamp—an uncontrolled situation. I am still not breathing. Janet, who has been held at a steady, moderate agony for about a minute now, asks through gasps, "What's wrong?"

Already the baby's losing too much blood and might bleed to death if the cord end isn't clamped soon. But how do you explain disaster while it's happening? Explanation interferes with resolution. There is a difference between studying a finished tombstone planted in a field and carving the names and dates on that tombstone. Dr. Wine's sedentary body only appears incapable of quick action, but after the initial shock, he recovers and calmly orders Janet to push hard. Why don't obstetricians just run away, screaming in terror?

The next enormous wave of pain crests on Janet's face. Other than windows, her face has always been the ultimate intended destination for my thoughts. Would telling her about the cord make this worse? When in the birthing room, where all roads lead to calm, do as the obstetricians do.

Wine says, "Push, yes, push." Janet's face turns quizzical, but then is seized by another pain surge. We tell the human to not push but the body is a contraption, it must complete its function. The body is furiously engaged in birth, its voice stronger than any doctor's.

Janet obeys. The body wanted this done, it was being prevented; now it can catch up. A single push and the rest of the baby's squeezed out. With the quickness of a cat in front of a mouse hole, Dr. Wine clamps the pulsatile, dangling cord. Then he dries the baby with a towel. After most of the clotty muck's removed, Dr. Wine places the nameless baby on the incubator. Most kids appear pink, hyperemic, but this one's pale, as bloodless as he is nameless. The nurse summons the neonatal team.

Wait. I am so afraid the baby might die that I haven't even acknowledged its sex. He. A boy. Master No Name.

It's been thirty seconds and the baby has yet to cry. I try to peek over the rising, falling, and sliding shoulders of the solo nurse. The kid is bluish-white, unmoving. A boy. "It's a boy, Janet," I say, not betraying concern. Will this baby live?

Janet, however, is happy, already transitioning from titanic pain to relief as if walking through a revolving door. Whoosh, ordeal over, deliverance. Besides, no one has informed her of the disaster yet.

The neonatal team arrives and begins their resuscitation dance. They lift, poke, rub, and attach. An old nurse, much esteemed in the medical faith, seems to be calling the shots with a grumpy impatience that is the perfect mirror of Dr. Wine—perhaps calm in this place is the gooey goodness inside a hard exterior? Only deep within are the necessary reserves, the strange substance that is leadership and experience, the saving amalgam. The old nurse projects an air that suggests she has performed thousands of these in the past, whereas a young member of the team, a female physician according to the dress code of shoe and coat, receives all of the nurse's barks. Each time she receives chastisement, the doctor responds, "Thank you." The Golden Rule is shared amongst most creeds but so is shaming, so is shunning. Abasement is necessary for some explorations in the medical faith.

Dr. Wine's hands are already clean, but he rubs them anyway on a blood-streaked towel as he watches the resuscitation. He has nothing to do with what happens now, the fate of the baby is literally out of his hands. He, too, has been released into the other side of the revolving door. In a short while, we hear our son's first cry. Dr. Wine's shoulders slightly fall, though he continues to dab his hands with the towel—he may not be responsible anymore, but he is still a learned part of the birth, implicated should that child stay blue. I note the window on the wall opposite Janet's head, one shielded by thick, socialist-style curtains. A small gleaming sliver shines through the middle.

Looking more closely: in the window sliver, I see a golden baby undergoing the Neonatal Resuscitation Protocol. Blotchy masked bodies apply positive pressure ventilation to the baby's face via a bag-valve-mask. An endotracheal tube is inserted. Chest compressions are started. Epinephrine is drawn up into a syringe.

"So what happened?" Janet says brightly while looking at the clump of bodies moving around the incubator. "I'd really like to know, if anyone could tell me." Janet, polite even in the middle of a disaster, as calm as any obstetrician. Janet, also like the obstetrician, is a surgeon. Both are about action, steadiness, resourcefulness—dealing with problems.

I'm about terror and imagination, about fearful fantasies projected onto windows. About hallucinations, or are they delusions? About fearing for the worst, preparing for the worst, and even though the disaster doesn't arrive, I expect the disaster to visit next time, that fear and preparation were necessary rituals to keep disaster at bay—anxiety as charm.

The old nurse murmurs something to Dr. Wine, who drops the towel and beckons me over to the incubator. As he hands me a pair of scissors, the clump of bodies around the incubator parts. A small swaddled body is there, a pink gift of the magi. Dr. Wine unwraps the baby and points close to the umbilicus. "You remember, right? Cut there."

The baby's chest rises, falls. He puffs small cries of protest at the cold, shaking his legs and arms in small oscillations. When I'm done, Dr. Wine readjusts the plastic clamp closer to the baby's body. There is a right and proper way, after all.

The resuscitation team laughs amongst themselves—everyone except the young doctor. The old nurse says, "Well, we didn't have to do much there, did we? But it was good practice all the same." When she says the word "practice," she turns her head and fixes on the young doctor.

"Thank you *so much*," the young doctor says with passion. "This was such a valuable learning experience." She reminds me of a kid called to the front of the class where the strap is used to leave a huge red welt across both hands, but the worst part of the experience for the child and the other students who witness the punishment is that the child must thank the teacher for the discipline.

Dr. Wine, having waited for the room to become more controlled and orderly, now encourages Janet to push out the placenta. "This is easy compared to before," he says. "Just a steady push, no need to strain."

As Janet pushes, he tells her what happened. An old doctor trick: while the patient is focused on something else, explain the disaster. There is great wisdom in this method because a direct approach is often misleading. Rendering bad news obliquely clears space for the message to sink in, making the information less inflicted than delivered. The placenta plops out, an eerie, oversized amoeba. "But everything is okay now," he concludes. "The baby perked up nicely at five minutes and that's really good. Because of the knot and the transection, we're going to have baby stay overnight in the neonatal unit. That probably isn't necessary but we like to be cautious. The first blood test will tell us everything. If the hemoglobin level is good, then baby's good." As he said this, Dr. Wine flipped the placenta over, appraising it like a diamond, ensuring completeness, that no parts are left behind in Janet.

Janet smiles as our wailing baby is handed to her. Dr. Wine's name is shouted from the other end of the birthing unit. Another incipient disaster unfolding down the hall summons his professional calm.

"Shane, this name just came to me when I felt his head popping out down there. Tell me, what do you think about 'Kazuo'?"

Our obstetrics nurse, busy mopping up blood, says, "Kazuo? So beautiful! What's that mean?"

"I'm half Japanese," Janet says, offering the missing connection. "So it's Japanese for 'man of peace.'"

Before Kazuo is wheeled away, I touch him over the front fontanelle. *Hi*, I think, extending the thought into his brain. I have no name and Janet already has a beautiful one. Cap slung over the right eye, giving the appearance of bepuzzlement, Kaz's blue left eye peeks out from his florid face—tranquillity in surrounding fire. *Rigel is Orion's blue suede shoe. Rigel is Orion's blue suede shoe.* Protect and shelter are the dual messages his body sends to me. His hands rise and his fingers curl as if he's touching himself after a dream.

Do we grow into our names eventually? Do our lives grow around our names, or despite them? My own name is strange to me, like a shorthand that never quite fits my shifting self. So close to shame, just one consonant removed, I've always felt like my name was called when someone said the word. Perhaps the false christening infected my own fatherhood, leaving me incapable of naming anything.

Next to my seat by Janet's bed is the naming book, kept close up to the last minute in the hopes it would finally offer up a name. Though I read every entry, none felt right. I flip the pages to "S", then to "Sh." The meaning of "Shane" is, apparently, "Graced by God."

Am I? I thought. *Have I been?*

Rather than razz me with "You better believe it!", BCJ hands me a stogie and we burn them down without anyone raising an objection. "Now you have a firstborn son, bro. *Heavy.*"

ENTER BURNING CROWN JESUS—ASK ME ANYTHING!

"We've received a load of questions this week from our audience, and we here at *Enter Burning Crown Jesus* are dedicated to listener service. We aim to satisfy you and make you feel as if you've been listened to, since you support us so well. Without your love and attention, we'd not have the privilege to be here and make this program. So, let's take them in order.

Why is it that complications always seem so tidy in retrospect? "In our previous program, we mentioned a balance between past experience and present experience, how the delusory mind tends to overvalue the immediate present. The truth is, all minds are delusory. They take events and make them self-referential as they occur. More, they imbue these events with meaning such that, when taken in toto, a person can feel as if they have purpose. Imagine if you could sort out the items in your house into two piles. In one pile, you are allowed only five things. Everything else goes into the other pile. The large pile is difficult to spin into a story. It is, in a way, *polythematic*, and lacks a commonality, a factor that can thread through the items and gather them into a larger narrative, other than the mere fact of them being there, on that particular day. The small pile, however, is quite likely *monothematic*. A picture of a little girl, almost three years old, in a silver frame, the little girl in a red dress with a red cap, hand on her hip, quizzical. A pink paperclip bent into the shape of an angel. A tinfoil halo. A book of poems titled *Open Up Your Heart*. A battered typescript of *Hamlet*. These items suggest a possible religiosity as well as paternity, and one can start to spin the yarn. Yet I would suggest to you that the owner of these—the person whose life has collected these items along its course, and selected them as the most significant artefacts of time—could write out an account of their importance in such personal terms that you might consider that soul deluded as to their actual worth. For, to anyone else, they are worthless."

Why is it that we never expect trouble until trouble occurs, and from that point on, complications are expected? "I see two answers to this. One is, mankind was cast out from the garden, so in actual fact, mankind was looking for trouble long before it occurred. I think the point important. The other answer probably connects more with the reason for your question. The listener knows he is paranoid, that paranoia is perhaps the most pervasive and intense element of his psychosis. Indeed, I can feel like something is jamming the broadcast at this point, that there is a self-sabotage in the listener himself. Paranoia calls the tune in Silly Shane's body; it is more powerful than even the god BCJ. I can say no more here, for fear of *Enter Burning Crown Jesus* being cancelled. And this show must go on."

Why do we invest meaning in events when they might be random? Why reach for fate or faith as explanations? "The first part of this has been answered already, which is of course a reflection of how our audience is repetitive and obsessed. But the second part is worth covering briefly, albeit in the form of a question, since the matter cannot be settled anyway. Listener, take your pick: the Divinely Ordained, God Works in Mysterious Ways Lemonade? Or, alternatively, Devil's Swill, the devil's will, the devil will, that nothing matters and meaning is only for those who choose delusion?"

What is the point of imperfect miracles? "As I have made you aware, I am into imperfection these days. I try to do a little good every once in a while, no more than once a day. I no longer try to convince people to act against their natures. I help a little old lady across the street. I take out an old man's garbage. I shovel out a driveway. Sure, I still tend to help the old the most, but that's only because they seem to need me more, perhaps even think of me more. It was a lot of trouble, once upon a time, seeking perfection. I'm rebranded: a Good Enough God."

BABY MONITOR

Burning Crown Jesus is in the gym, working shoulders and lats. The prince of peace sweats all over the equipment, failing to wipe it down. A neglectful god. "This is a metaphor," BCJ says.

"What is a metaphor? The gym, for the temple of my body?"

"No, silly. This is how your illness is always doing pushups, waiting for you in the parking lot."

"But you are not my illness," I say. "And now that's a mixed metaphor."

Jesus says nothing, as occupied as he is at the squat rack. Down quick, slow up cycle—perfect form. The gym is now crowded with dozens of other sweating bodies, all taking turns on occupied machines.

Jesus is pretty ripped. He could be the next cover model for *Men's Health*. "I think we need to have a talk. You're not getting this."

Oh oh.

"Why am I only here when you need me? Why am I a kind of on-call emergency rescue worker for you? I'm showing you the gym. This is where you could grow stronger in the faith, and not need me to save your ass whenever you're in a jam." Jesus strikes a pose and just gives 'er, a superflexing man of steel.

Tough love. But the old kind wasn't working. I get it. I ignored Jesus, I wouldn't let him save me. He's changing tactics. "Okay, Jesus. No more trips to the Land O Gulps. From now on, the Sweat Shop."

AFTER SPENDING SIX MONTHS IN HOSPITAL post-plummet, too ill to complete my residency in emergency medicine in Halifax, I took care of Zee during her third year of life. Unable to work as a doctor or to take care of myself, I nevertheless was entrusted with the most important task of all: daily responsibility for my daughter.

That long series of days acquainted me with Zee's three-ness: a fierce exploratory energy, inquisitive intelligence, and unending quest for cookies. I am loathe to metaphorize my child as an antidepressant, but the truth is that without the purpose her needs constituted, as well as the perpetually refreshed joy she brought to life, I wouldn't be alive. Wake up; breakfast; chore; morning activity; television; lunch; nap; afternoon activity; supper; television; bedtime; repeat. I trod this schedule every day, trailing behind a comet. I took care of her, but in doing so, she really took care of me.

We moved to Guelph because Janet, who has always wanted to be a veterinarian, has been accepted to Ontario Veterinary College, but also because the city has a psychiatric hospital that specializes in the treatment of physicians.

To the east side of our apartment complex, a chain-link fence fronts gnarled trees that bear a minimum of leaves in the summer. I'm not sure what the landscape architect students were thinking. The see-through border does little to protect the interior from observation. Choking tendrils that snake up from the ground attract clinging snow, giving the trees a soft, downy look in the winter. In the summer, long grass pencils up. Fellow dwellers often tip their large household items over this low fence. Motorists passing by might conclude that the junk is protected from the inhabitants of Wellington Woods and not the other way around.

One afternoon, as part of our daily walkabout, Zee and I notice a newly abandoned leather car seat gleaming behind the fence. Though the cushion is missing, we could still use it to play Ghost Car. Or Rocket Ship. Though there's a new thing, she'll probably want to play Trashy Game. Just as I benefit from the safe orbit provided by routines, so do children.

"Daddy, *Trashy*."

The garbage heap Oracle known as Trashy is her favourite character from the Jim Henson show *Fraggle Rock*. Trashy sees the future but renders it obscurely to characters doomed to grasp her prophecies only in retrospect. When Trashy finishes prophesying in the vowel roundedness and off glide of the New York accent, Jewish matriarch version, two rat acolytes state in unison, "Trash Heap Has Spoken. Meaaaah."

I mangle an attempt to sound like Trashy. Luckily, the key to the performance is less aural and more structural: one must make a mysterious opening statement. That way, an open system is created. Zee can take the story whatever way she wants to go, which is important because Zee understands stories and prefers to make her own.

"You cannot leave the magic," I intone, each word spoken slowly, moaningly.

"What magic?" she asks skeptically, hand on her hip, elbow cocked. Classic Zee.

"All the junk on the other side of the fence. New stuff. New *magic*. You cannot leave the magic."

"Okay, Trashy, we can go Trashy! Daddy—Trashy—lift me."

I lift Zee over. She cursorily explores this world of lost refrigerators and split dishwashers, eyes wide, until she finally finds the new addition. "Trashy, this. This, Trashy."

Someone walks down the sidewalk limning Stone Road. "Daddy, you come now. You come now."

I lever myself over the fence and let Zee direct me to do and say whatever she wants. Now Zee is Trashy, sitting atop a broken car seat throne, and I'm one of her rat attendants. She tells a fortune involving a frosted cinnamon roll at the Tim Hortons about a kilometre away. A prophecy involving cookies. Smart girl. "Magic sugar. *Maaaaaaaaaagic*." Trashy really can tell the future. Being on this side of the fence, we're that much closer to the donut shop.

ONE NIGHT I BRING THE BABY MONITOR OUT OF RETIREMENT, placing it on the ledge above Kaz's bed. The monitor's green light forms a focal point in the room. I want to redeem this good light, to be on the side of order, to say that the glow makes the room safer, but the tint is nauseating, sickly—enough to make me look jaundiced.

My large bedroom window opens onto a view of Victory Public School where a motion-activated sensor triggers a powerful playground-bathing light. Whenever the wind blows, the sensor activates, triggering twenty seconds of illumination. When well, I often look out the window and try to see if an animal or errant bouncy ball triggered the sensor, a shape rolling or scampering near the fence. When unwell, I interpret the light as if it were Morse code. Two close firings is a dash, but one alone with some space on either side is a dot. No need to record the dots and dashes tonight, though, I already know the universe's message: *not right.*

The streetlight fires again, feels like snow shining up from below. For a short time, everything in the room is visible, the green blessedly gone, only a white cleansing light.

MY STORY IS NOT ONE OF LINEAR, INCREMENTAL PROGRESS. Think of it more like the dots and dashes of Morse code, the intervals between words, the pauses between caller and respondent. BCJ appears, a conversation ensues, time passes, BCJ returns, dot dash dot pause, BCJ racks up frequent flyer points.

BCJ is a miracle worker but even miracles have their limits. It took time to find a community doctor in Guelph capable of listening—Dr. Pink. Not all psychiatrists have the capability. "It would make sense that you have bipolar disorder," she says, "given your family history and the fact that olanzapine has been of some help. Would you be willing to start on lithium?"

If only I told Pink about BCJ, the diagnosis would be so much easier. But if I told Pink about BCJ, then god would lose his cover, and the end of my professional career would be nigh.

Lithium is the drug that the poet Robert Lowell used, one that kept him out of hospitals for a long, long time. At one point in his life, before he was introduced to lithium, he was admitted at least once a year. Lowell is a hero of mine. He wrote beautiful things about Harriet, his daughter.

"Okay," I say.

I CAN'T SLEEP. Adapted Nietzsche: If you listen to the baby monitor, the baby monitor also listens to you. The logic is simple: the future watcher tells himself, *My child mustn't die while I am on duty.* But all guardianship can only ever be partial. The guardian needs to sleep too, yet the need for watching is perpetual. This is the unresolvable paradox.

I listen to my son's breathing as reassurance he is still alive but also because it soothes me to hear him breathe. When Kaz turns away from the receiver, or when his blankets rustle, an alarm triggers and I wake. If I don't hear rhythmic breathing soon, I check to find him sleeping comfortably, turned from the monitor, soft blankie on the floor, his arms and legs dangling off the edge of the bed.

Back to bed. Back to the baby monitor's small, static hiss lying underneath a relay of rhythmic breathing. Back to the cycle: I either can't hear Kaz breathe or I convince myself that I can't, making me concentrate harder, and soon either Kaz breathes more loudly or reception picks up again. This listening begins to infect my dreams, where I dream of listening and not hearing, so I wake to hear breathing sounds. I dream of waking up and not hearing breathing sounds, thus I get up and check again. Checking. Checking, checking, checking. Hiss, a snake in the room, in the dark, in my dreams.

Sleep is necessary I tell myself. Unlike the baby monitor, I don't listen. Machines are badly out of alignment. Mechanisms are wearing on themselves. In my dreams, I lift his little body up and place him on my lap, his limbs loose. I want my son back. Give him back.

So drained by the watching, so exhausted. I am such a philistine, so ungrateful. BCJ is always there, committed, whereas I outsource the process to technology. *There is no perfection*, I tell myself. BCJ appears in the window opposite, a brief flash in the white light from the playground, his thumb up.

ZEE IS ONLY THREE YEARS OLD, a perfect three. A few days ago, I had picked her up and said, "You are not allowed to get older. You must always stay three! Stay three forever!"

But when I put her down, she stamped her right foot and defiantly said, "I growing, Daddy. I growing!"

With a wide stance, blue net choked too high at the neck, Zee charges in pursuit of butterflies, falling, getting up, chasing, waving, enthralled, determined to catch a beautiful insect herself. We spend hours in a groundhog-holed field adjacent to Wellington Woods. Zee runs and swings her net until she's exhausted, eventually handing it off to me to capture her quarry. When I catch one, she dances, peers at it in the net, and then solemnly opens her hand. This is the signal to carefully extricate the creature and then place it on her finger. Watching it fly away, she says, "We're not hurting them, are we Daddy?"

"No," I lie. "We're introducing them to us!" Hand on hip, Zee seems skeptical. I tell another lie: "Trashy will show the butterflies how to get back to the field."

In time, Zee asks if we can keep some of the butterflies we catch, but only the ones she classifies as "good." Science lesson: I punch holes in the top of a peanut butter container and teach Zee about habitats. Each day we make a new one, refreshing the greenery inside. I buy Zee an Ontario-based bugopedia so she can learn names like the Silver-Spotted Skipper, Black Swallowtail, and Cabbage White. She's permitted three butterflies every hunt. "One bug for every year you are old," I explain.

I put the jar on a shelf that Zee can spot but not reach. She checks on her catch several times a night, the light in her room turning on and off. When she wakes up, the first thing we do together is open the jar near the junk lot to let the insects escape. After breakfast, we'll refresh the jar and plan the next bug hunt.

"When I four, I have four butterflies?" she says, counting on her fingers.

A year later, Groundhog Field becomes a construction site that spawns a sprawling big-box shopping complex. In the early stages as equipment accumulated, the groundhogs seemed spooked, their holes un-popped out of. But in just a few days, the holes were smoothed over by bulldozers and then capped with asphalt. Hopefully they weren't buried alive.

Seven years later, during the time Zee fell ill, I buy her a pink bike helmet at the Canadian Tire that now rests on Groundhog Field. "Zee, do you remember chasing butterflies here?" I ask.

"In the store?" she asks. Zee has no memory of where she once stood.

"We used to come right here, where we are standing now, and I followed after you as you ran around and tried to catch butterflies. A giant field! All dirt and grass! And *groundhogs*."

"Nope. Wasn't this always a Canadian Tire?" she asks, expressionless.

The memory is worth fighting for. "Remember the day you turned four? The first thing you wanted to do was go to Groundhog Field and get four butterflies. We even put an extra hole in the top of the habitat, for extra butterfly breathing."

I still pass by this section of heavily-developed city tucked against the Hanlon Parkway on the way to and from work. The feeling is: it's as if we were never there, that it's impossible we ever were. Twice a day, I try to convince myself the experience is simply one of pleasant reminiscence. Twice a day, I fail. The actual process is mourning.

KAZ FALLS TO THE FLOOR AND CONVULSES. Janet rushes to her son. As she has been instructed, she marks the time: 10:07 AM, T0. She works a blanket under his head. She turns him on his side into the recovery position. And she waits.

Question: How long should one wait when one's son is shaking on the floor? Answer: the rotating cast of physicians told us five minutes, but immediately if he turns blue. The boy, on a blanket, removed from this world. How many times have we told Kaz to wait just a moment for the things he wants, admonishing him, *It's almost here! Just wait five more minutes, you can do it!*

Janet calls the ambulance at T5. So far, he has not become Little Boy Blue.

Boys dressed as paramedics arrive at T11. Though they attach the monitors to Kaz's vibrating chest expertly, they seem uncomfortable at the acuity of the call. "Get the level threes here," one of them says to dispatch through the radio on his vest. In the squawk, I can distinguish the dispatcher issuing coordinates to a different team of paramedics.

What is a level three? Janet hovers over our jerking little boy as the paramedics affix an oxygen mask. They try to use an elastic band to get their hands free, but Kaz's motion keeps jostling the mask off.

Janet kneels near Kaz's head, murmuring as she rubs his hair. I can't hear what she's saying—I'm too loud, whispering *BE OK BE OK BE OK*. Kaz's breath isn't audible, so I focus on Janet's impromptu lullaby, *something Kazzy something something Kazzy love something Kazzy . . . .*

At thirteen minutes in, the seizure still has not stopped. The two younglings try to pry open Kaz's mouth with an oral airway, but his jaw's too clenched. If anything, they're damaging his teeth. One of the indistinguishable monitor-sticker-on-ers touches his radio.

Ten minutes now—the system's requisite period of negligent waiting. This feels like my childhood, when I stared for hours on end at a ceramic manger, the three wise men surrounding Mary and her baby. In a small Guelph kitchen, a mother, a father, and two strangers watch a small boy.

Blood drips from Kaz's mouth onto the kitchen floor. Since the short seizure at the daycare, Kaz has had a handful of additional small ones. This is the most violent seizure Kaz has ever had. His body thrums, then gyrates. Blood puddles under his head, smearing his neck, but then a big convulsion lifts him up and smashes his cheek into the blood.

At T18, a second ambulance pulls in directly behind an already parked one. Disaster math: one little boy = two ambulances? Heavy-set, middle-aged men bearing the burden of pudgy, weary experience amble out of the second ambulance. They waddle to the back of their bus, pull out bags of drugs and implements. Ruddy and Tall saunter in from the street as the slow sweet arrival of release, the casual promise of help. Do we, the people in need, have to wait to be helped? Do we have to earn help by waiting? Is waiting an essential process of deserving help? And for help to be effective, does our need have to increase to the point of desperation?

Ruddy says to Tall, "They got the rescue board in there, right?" Tall responds, "Yeah. They did that at least. Ma'am, move back please." They shift Kaz for transport. I'm already well back, very far away. *The driver on the bus says move back please, move back please, move back please....* Ruddy and Tall have already drawn up drugs on the way over. Maybe preparation needs to take its time? Maybe one can't force cure. The ruddy one snakes a tube up my son's nose and injects liquid into the tube. The tall one pries an airway device past Kaz's teeth-clench. Then the ruddy one transfers my son onto a rescue board set out by the useless younger team that's watching as helplessly as I am. Though Kaz is rigid and writhing, the giant man turns him gently, sliding the board underneath. The paramedics lift the board, place it onto a roller, and pull straps around Kaz's body.

Kaz has been down for nineteen minutes now.

His body slows, the limb spasms becoming bigger and longer. One of the young paramedics contacts triage at the Guelph General. "Looks like midaz is working," he says into his vest comm. The ruddy one smirks at him as if to say, *Yeah, we handle shit.*

The seizure defiantly resumes its original amplitude. The useful paramedics take head and foot, while the useless ones man Kaz's flanks. They carry him like pallbearers to the waiting ambulance without urgency, all the people in need of help thinking *faster, faster* while those in the helping professions know that steady competence wins the race. Does the same go for religion, the slow self-save that brings about an eventual, graduated realization that, in fact, the supplicant is exactly where he needs to be?

Once Kaz is secured by straps and clips, the paramedics join the ranks of us mere watchers. Who can heal the child? Somehow, a stuffy is in my hand. I must have walked upstairs as the drama was unfolding and found Harambe somewhere in Kaz's room. Next to Kaz's shaking head, I place the gorilla stuffy, soon vibrating to Kaz's frequency.

DR. PINK'S SMALL OFFICE in the Homewood psychiatric hospital keeps moving around, just like the groundhogs once did. When I ask her why, she smiles ruefully and says the owners of the facility are chicken farmers who bring just-in-time supply and maintenance principles to hospital operations. I can only infer that these principles extend to physician management.

Her ritual invocation: "How have things gone since I saw you last?"

My ritual response: "I don't know. You'll have to tell me."

That's true enough: I *never* know. Before jumping from a rooftop, I could be asked that question and have the same answer. The difficulty is that I feel poorly all the time, which means there are no dynamics to permit distinguishing affective states. When is too hot, too hot? I possess an energy that is boundless, uncontainable, inexhaustible, one that needs to be directed to a productive activity else it consumes me.

"Maybe it's better if I ask you more obvious things. How is your sleep?"

"Five hours a night. But broken." Attention's challenged too—I hear the waiting room's muzak playing on a tinny speaker through the door of Pink's office.

"How is your concentration?"

"Intact." Still talking like a doctor.

"Are you having thoughts of killing yourself?"

Tell the truth? Don't tell the truth? "Not exactly. Though I hear this constant thought through my mind: *I hate my life I hate my life I hate my life.*"

"That's an intrusive thought. How does it make you feel?"

"It's embarrassing."

"Why?"

"It means I'm weak. I shouldn't think this way."

"Why?"

"I'm alive. I have a wife and daughter, things I never thought I would have. I have nothing to complain about."

Bidden now, the intrusive thoughts initiate their program: *I hate my life I hate my life I hate my life.* I try to push the thoughts out to a tiny rectangular window in the lower right section of the posterior wall, but they won't go.

"Maybe it's information, a signal. What else happened this month?"

TODAY FEATURES ONLY ONE OBJECTIVE: Zee and I are going to build a snowman. Snowman Artisan Zee blurts all at once: "We-need-eyes-

and-ears-and-mouth-and-carrot!" Upon investigation, the refrigerator offers a good selection: carrot nose, two eye onions, a beet mouth, and two ear leaves ripped from a romaine lettuce. Outside, we easily scavenge two willow twigs for arms. "This snowman is going to be me!" she says. Zee looks over at the fence where imaginary Trashy lives. "Next day we build a snow *family*, Daddy?"

"Sure, Zee. Tomorrow we build Mommy Snow, Daddy Snow, even Snow Cat."

The wet quickly packs into solid, large balls. Uninterested in making the balls herself, Snowman Artisan Zee supervises the construction process. "Put roll-y circles here, Daddy!" In addition to supervisor, she's also the details girl, poised to make the face. She sticks the carrot deep into the head; other vegetables are placed at Picasso angles. The beet mouth gives Snow Zee the appearance of wearing purple lipstick. "Good snowman," she judges, flopping onto a footprint-free area of our backyard, waving her arms and legs to make an angel. As she flails, pigments bleed out of the beet, down the snowman's chin and onto her belly.

Tomorrow I might be too exhausted to want to play. To dispel this thought, I mock-run from Zee, pretending to be afraid. Our old standby, the faithful favourite of my fatherhood. "Chase Game!" she screams. We have the whole day to stalk the backyard, more than enough time to tire her out and go inside, peel off her sopping snowsuit, and put her to bed for a nap. But it only takes an hour. "Too big for naps. Too big," she protests, against reason. In a minute, her glare shifts gradually into acquiescence, and then is soon traded for the glaze of a not uncharitable dreamland.

A solution comes to the problem of tomorrow's unpredictability. While Zee sleeps, I return to the backyard to make Snow Cat, the quickest job; then a svelte Snow Mommy; Snow Daddy comes last, made far from the site of the family because the easy, proximate snow got used during construction of the other snow family members. I roll his big boulder components to the family scene, parts crumbling off with motion. Tomorrow, details girl can decorate the faces of the promise I kept.

BECAUSE I CAN'T TELL HOW I'M FEELING and can only gauge second-arily, by how much I'm *doing*, I am further down the line of impending disaster than some others are before they seek help. This means that I see Dr. Pink on a regular basis as a surveillance measure. She's there to tell me if I'm well or not. I'm supposed to be there to listen.

The problem is my energy, which either magnifies extremely or dis-sipates to the point where I don't want to get out of bed. Almost always in both contexts, I have been able to work and see patients as a way to get out of myself and to focus on someone else. Interviewing other people provides a wonderfully predictable structure, which is part of its restorative power.

Outside the office, where there is less structure, where expectations are not as regimented, where I'm writing poems about how much it hurts to be a vulnerable human being—*how much* I'm doing can easily get lost in *what* I'm doing. Once upon a time, I got quite lost and the last step I took was off a balcony.

It's been six long months of not working, of not being able to go to the oasis of other people to help them. Dr. Pink and I meet in a differ-ent office, this time in the Hamilton end of the building. Construction debris and caution tape litter the hallway passage. She dubs her new digs "The Dungeon." Truly, it's the worst working space she's yet had in the institution. I imagine a lullaby playing over the hospital PA, all the doctors playing musical offices, the doctors waylaid in hallways and banished when the music stops.

"You seem somewhat sped-up right now. I think we should go a little higher on the medication," Dr. Pink says.

I don't want to. Not at all. *But I'm not gibbering. I'm not drooling. The tinfoil remains untouched in the kitchen drawer.* "Okay," I say.

"But before we talk about that, are you aware of anything else hap-pening in your life, any other stress?"

"I wish I was back at work. I love helping other people."

"That's good, but you're not well enough to go back to work right now."

"I know. This is a lament."

"Let's consider other things. How's your family?"

"They're fine. If I had to guess, all the fluctuation is probably due to all the shit I had to go through as a kid. I'm not sure it's possible to get over that."

DELHI STREET IS HARDLY A HILL by the Lake of Galilee, but this is my Sermon on the Mount nevertheless. I walk up the incline to the hospital. For the second time in my life, I am placed in restraints, although this time the bindings are to the sky.

Why run? The lesson shown thus far is to take my time, to be patient. Snow too white for the scene suffocates the suburban lawns, spilling out onto the road. Yet there is no cloud above that could be a culprit. I bawl like I did as a kid, when I could be hurt in a way that was permanent, that sponsors every step I take. My father's face blocks out the sky.

I look up and beg, "Please let him live. I'll do anything, anything, if you let him live."

The bindings at my wrists tug again, cinching tighter. In the elevated distance, I see small shapes re-enter an ambulance, possibly to competence the fuck out of another slow-motion emergency. They drive further up the hill and out of sight. My wrists and ankles strangulate, each step drawing the celestial drawstring tighter. Is my son alive? I need to touch him, lay my hands on him and speak a word in his ear. Suddenly that's all the praying I want to do.

ZEE FIGURE SKATES AT EXHIBITION ARENA just a short walk from our house. She wears a red dress that once was worn by Janet from when she skated as a child. Tensed pose, arms upraised, she is almost totally extended. A note she wrote me in careful pencil contains the individual program elements in sequence:

Start with right hand on heart, toe pick in ice. Left outside three turn, back cross, lunge, back cross, right foot back, back cross X2, waltz jump, skate wavy on right foot, fan lick with left foot, flip jump, toe bob, Mohawk, cross, cross, cross, camel spin, sit spin, back spin, cross, cross, cross, spiral

for 7 seconds, Mohawk, cross, cross, cross, cross, Lutz jump,
loop, Mohawk, cross, Mohawk, Salchow, three turn, cross,
cross, cross, flip jump, cross, three turn, lunge, cross, Lutz
jump, three turn, corkscrew spin, jump cross, spinny thing
with right foot going around and left toe pick in ice, arms
over the head and then they slowly fall down.

Around her, blue, pink, purple, and green-dressed girls spin like gaseous
atoms careening about the ice—Brownian motion made elegant. Before
a likely crash, one skater inevitably softens a turn or changes direction
to find a free patch of ice. Skaters practise for two-hour sessions three
times a week in an effort to perfect their routines: how to flawlessly land
a series of jumps, spins, and stylish spirals. They spend hours striding
and falling out there, learning how to move with grace and power. Older
girls attempt double axels and double toe loops. A girl close to Zee's age
works on a flying camel spin. Younger girls gleefully shoot the duck and
laugh when they fall.

The Guelph Figure Skating Club coaches dress in black jackets and
yoga pants, pointing, nodding, alternatingly making stern then encouraging faces. Billing in fifteen-minute blocks, they draw sinuous lines on
the ice with bingo dabbers and shout advice. *Head up head up keep your
line* Coach J admonishes. Vince the Zamboni Man moves from the back
garage to the front rink office, rubbing the cigarette pack in his front
shirt pocket as girls stretch on the boards, their legs lifted over the top
as if scrambling over a fence.

Zee dips down, working on her flexibility; girls fatigued from hard
skating move to the boards to prop themselves up, feigning to stretch,
catching their breath to talk to one another, sucking in the dry air and
giving back their hydration to the atmosphere; other girls drink from
their water bottles, having respirated too much of the rink air. Girls in
groups of twos and threes stand at the north and south ends of the ice,
laughing about something other than figure skating.

Zee runs through her routine as I lean closer to the high window in
the arena's viewing room, twenty feet up. Her right pick strikes the ice

and she's into the flip jump, vertical, crossing distance, revolving. Her red practice dress fans out like an open parasol, a red Zee amidst the rink's softer sworl of pinks, peaches, light blues. Just a half-second in the air, she holds her arms close as she touches down to make a fluid push forward, arms reaching out for accentuation. She's moving now to her program's final element, gaining speed to conclude with a spin that stops in her starting position. As she's been taught, she dramatically lifts her head, waiting a moment to open her eyes and then, a beat later, to mechanically smile.

I wave at her, try to catch her attention, but she doesn't see me. When the lesson's over, and we're walking home in the winter dark, Zee says, "J. said for me to practise smiling, so that I can do it when I have to in competitions. To improve my performance."

I have stared in the mirror and never found a real smile, long sessions in which the human is never verified, BCJ popping in and out in the background, holding a placard with self-affirmation slogans. I am successful. I am confident. I am getting better and better every day. I am an unstoppable force of nature.

Maybe you, BCJ. Maybe you.

BCJ AND I ARE CHILLIN' AT THE WALMART MCDONALD'S, trying to solve the secrets of faith, just rappin' about life and love and the meaning of here and now, the vagaries of time, with only the occasional digression into stock market trading intricacies, when Jesus interrupts our comparison of mythologies and says, "Bro. I gots to get me some TRIPLE FUDGE."

"Triple Fudge? McDonald's sells fudge, like the kind you bake in ovens?"

"No, bro." He stands, and beckons to the counter. "Follow me, and I shall make you a fisher of fudge."

We walk past all the retired dudes discoursing on finasteride and prostates, on the relative merits of different phosphodiesterase blockers—what romantic situations are best for which, you gotta get your money's worth—and how atrophic vaginitis is a real bitch for guys. At the counter, an androgynous teenager with purple hair and a nametag declaring "Onyx" stands behind the register. "What can I get for you?"

BCJ, who is smiling as if the practice is free, says, "I needs me a hot fudge sundae, but with triple fudge. Not single, not double, but triple. *Triple*. Got that?"

"Okay, sir. Got it." She moves to the ice cream dispenser. Smiles are no longer free on Jesus's face. Smiles are expensive, are part of an austerity regime. Jesus is inspecting wares, is determining if works are real, if a soul is worth saving. Jesus stares at Onyx.

First, the bottom layer of fudge. Single. Then, ice cream, shoved out somehow by hydraulics, a white goo stream, circles laid down in the cup. Then, a top layer of fudge. As Onyx puts a lid on the container, Jesus judges.

"That is not TRIPLE FUDGE! That is DOUBLE FUDGE and I asked for TRIPLE! TRIPLE FUDGE!"

Mortifyingly, BCJ turns to me. "See how they always only do double fudge when ya ask for triple fudge? Always only double, even though you get them to say triple before they start the pour! I mean, what's so hard about making a fucking hot fudge sundae. TRIPLE! Do I have to show them how to do it? Do I have to do it myself? I always have to do everything myself!"

Onyx rapidly transforms the sundae into the realm of quintuple fudge, blackness flowing over the sides of the top. Handed the sundae, Jesus is impressed. "Onyx, I didn't know you had it in you. This is the greatest sundae in history. I shall remember you, Onyx, I shall remember you."

Onyx looks so rattled, they forget to make BCJ pay. "Want some?" he asks me, licking his spoon.

A MONITOR FOR HOW I'M DOING would sound like this: *Hissssssss.*

Janet and I sit across from one another, a distance magnified by the lack of a bed. "Kaz seized the whole way here. There were so many people ready. Nurses held him. They got an IV. They gave him something, I don't know what. They connected him to a monitor. His breathing got worse. The seizure didn't stop but he breathed too shallow, they said, so they bagged him. They had to help him breathe. He couldn't do it on his own anymore."

I have sharpened my prayer to perfection: *BE OK BE OK BE OK.*

Other people hear me, look, and then resolutely look away. The only distinction between myself and the mad whisperer on the streetcorner or ward is that the nightmare infesting my field of view is real.

A strange competition in my brain: a wild concern for my son versus self-consciousness, the effect I'm having on other people. Kaz's breath cannot be heard amidst the din of medical implement and busyness. Like when he was born, I can see him only in snippets as yellow-gowned bodies circulate around the bed. Unable to use his breath as anchor, I resolve to use the whispering against itself.

Each second contains one *BE OK*, each minute, sixty *BE OKs*. Five *BE OKs* elapse during oxygen mask placement; forty during monitor attachment; it takes seventy-four for the second IV insertion and flow. Somewhere in the bag of normal saline is the saving substance, a molecular structure with few drug-drug interactions, low protein-binding and low lipophilicity, that crosses the blood-brain barrier in a flash and sings lullabies to neurons, *Hush little baby don't say a word.*

BE OK BE OK BE OK.

This kind of counting isn't working. Now slowed from continuous flow, I try counting the drips from the bag. Although regularly timed, the interval between drips is a little over a second. This works—the whispering slows, then stops. The IV pole is jostled by one of the nurses setting out an intubation kit on the bed. The bag swings slightly. Stuck to its uppermost portion is a fat strip of orange tape bearing the handwritten name of the drug: *BE OK.*

AT THE MICROPHONE, Burning Crown Jesus looks distressed. "Hurry the fuck up and sit down, I'm about ready to do this shit," he says. His eyes are wild, he waves a sheaf of papers in one hand, a cellphone in the other. "It's POETRY TIME." The bookstore audience, previously milling about, looks confused. Since when do bookstore patrons rush to seat themselves at poetry readings?

"NOW!" Burning Crown Jesus screams, and the audience does as commanded. They turn to the rickety metal chairs and plant themselves, an obedient yet nonplussed crowd of downwardly mobile millennials, all fighting the power, all dependent on parental sinecures, all poets themselves.

"I need some fucking water," BCJ yells to the proprietor, a meek woman in the back named Janelle. "Janelle. Yo. The Jesus whistle needs wettin'."

Somehow Janelle is prepared for this part of the mass. A water bottle crowdsurfs to BCJ, buffeted up and down by hands. BCJ accepts the water aggrievedly, as if he must be grateful but wants to make a point at the same time, as if this gift should have been foreordained, ready. "Thanks," he says sharply, and then mutters something that sounds like *fucketyfucketyfuckety*, an obscene doxology. The papers in his hand go through a wild resequencing, as if the poems are out of order, or are instead missing something critical. *Fucketyfucketyfuckety.*

He screws the cap off the bottled water, chugs it halfway, and then coughs. He sticks out his tongue towards the ceiling, as if he might be testing the taste of the air, or perhaps wind direction, and coughs again. *Fucketyfucketyfuckety.* Another big draught on the water. Tongue vertical again. *Fucketyfucketyfuckety.*

Then he paces at the front, though he has only three feet of clearance on either side in the small store. BCJ is muttering to himself again, but this time about the Jews, international banking systems, and lies. He might walk all day, escaping Herod, until he suddenly stands still. "This one is for my fans," he says, in dulcet tones, nary a trace of the previous vocal raspiness, the threatened imperfections no longer auguring a marred performance. "And my fans, they are unvaxxed, right? No voluntary admittance of microchips to the lifestream, we are purebloods, *we* refuse to do the bidding of Pfizer. I have the best fans. *You.*" His head drops.

"GOTTERDAMMERUNG!" he suddenly screams, facing the crowd down. "GOTTERDAMMERUNG!" And then he stands back, pleased with this performance.

A small child in the audience starts to cry. Perhaps a year old, the babe lies in its mother's lap. The young woman tries to silence the child by breastfeeding, but the child won't latch, the crying won't stop. Either not a poetry fan, not religious, or merely hungry, the child is having some kind of crisis or temptation of the flesh.

Fucketyfucketyfuckety. Jesus tries to overwhelm the child's cries, cannonading a poem about the beauty of the universe and the somnolence of snowflakes, somehow disturbingly related to a nefarious network of greedy Jewry and Jewishness and *fucketyfucketyfuckety,* but before he finishes his ode, he singles out the woman, his face now frothing, spittle spinning out of the cosmos of his carious mouth. "Bringing a baby to a reading. *Fucketyfucketyfuckety.* A baby. A fucking baby! That baby is interfering with my greatness! The baby is crying on purpose. FUCK BABIES, fuck that baby and FUCK ALL BABIES."

The woman, carrying her baby, flees.

"GOTTERDAMMERUNG!" he says to the bookstore's closing glass door, pumping his fist. "TUSKFUCK!"

Why are the clothes of Jesus so soiled, thick with dirt, almost petrified? Why does Jesus smell like a garbage can? *Walk worthy of the vocation wherewith ye are called.*

With a final *fucketyfucketyfuckety,* the Christ moves through a crowd still too polite to leave the poor homeless person's recitation of doggerel, and picks up an empty chair, throwing it across the store. And lo, the hipsters finally flee.

MOTIONLESS FOR AN HOUR, Kaz sleeps in a place where his spirit can't be found. The parental stages of waiting for his return are numerous and cruel: first, we wait for the seizure to stop; then we wait for him to wake up; then we wait to see if he has been damaged somehow by the uncontrolled and prolonged seizure; then we wait for the next one to take him away again. Each stage has its own intensity, moving from hate into a decrescendo of chronic wariness.

Until recently, I've walked the hallways of the Guelph General Hospital with the dual identities of both patient and doctor. Now I have a third, that of average father, and this identity outranks the others. New on the scene, it immediately takes command.

In my experience, every patient or parent wants something, be it diagnosis, relief, escape, or sometimes just simple human interaction. Much has been written about the power of skin to skin contact after a baby is born to a mother, but the principle holds true for the rest of our lives, even if we largely give up skin for voice as we grow into adulthood. For a doctor practising modern biomedicine, the clinical exam is supposed to gather information, be a tool. But we must also acknowledge its dual identity: despite the cover provided by modern medical trappings, talking to patients is always the shaman's turn to enter into Western medicine: I touch, therefore I am, to you; and you are, to me. Though we are uncomfortable admitting the case, the same relation goes for parents and children who informally examine each other with hugs, pats, and squeezes that constitute one of the languages of love. There is something beyond us when we are together, with one another.

Scientific medicine cannot quantify this quality, and so it gives nothing to the patient or family except information, cure, or palliation. Happening parallel to conventional medical practice, though, is shamanism—the strange relational factor that freights the news, that delivers the pill. *Believe*, says the shaman. And if patients don't believe because the shaman refuses his nature and prefers to hide behind aseptic scientific or evidence-based practice, then patients will suffer for that lack.

We are not supposed to blame our gods. To grow spiritually, we are supposed to hold ourselves accountable. But for some of us, the conditions for faith have never been laid. To be a good shaman, I have stood over the bodies of sick and dying children as if I were not a doctor, but a parent.

Consider this kind of poem composed at the bedside of my son: nurses watch Kaz, tending to feebly protesting monitors though there's no alarm for cure, only for problem, error, and catastrophe. The living we are cheated of, and the dead are what we remember of beauty. How long have we been sitting here? Janet is asleep. Kaz—still sleeping.

"Mr. Neilson. Kazuo's admitted now. Any questions?"

I don't know what to ask anymore, since there aren't answers anyway. Asking and answering are like monsters under the bed: children who peek are asking for it.

ON A WALL DISPLAY AT VICTORY PUBLIC SCHOOL, a hundred crayoned pictures feature dogs and peace, friends and peace, swimming pools and peace, trees and peace, baseball diamonds and peace. According to the framing display prompt, "Peace Is ... whatever you think it is. Students, draw it!" Zee's picture depicts a storm-tossed ocean, black and mordant blue. The roiling ocean has a quality of sound, the crayons conjure a synesthetic roar. An observer feels viscerally placed in the scene.

My thoughts begin to extend to her picture because her ocean seems to me like a liquid window. Did the teacher wonder at the contrast between this picture of violent ocean and its overhanging sliver of horizonal sky, distinguished from its peers by an absence of friends, dogs and bicycles? Positioned amongst surrounding conventional colours, did the teacher worry the way my thoughts do as they extend to the picture?

TWO HOURS SINCE THE THIRTY-MINUTE-LONG SEIZURE STOPPED, my son still hasn't moved. What did the scan show? Frank Sinatra capers across my vision, top hat on, singing "A few more hours, that's all the time I got." Kaz's left leg shifts. Janet squeezes my hand; she sees it too. In a few minutes his face slides into the familiar agonized contortion, attesting to the beating his brain self-administered earlier. What he just went through is like an unfit adult completing an Ironman triathlon.

Janet's cheeks seem pulled down, somehow, as if weighted, her eyes more inset, dimmer, the opposite of my irradiating fire. I wrap my arms around her. I know what despair is like.

"They bagged him," she repeats. "A big paramedic asked me to step back. They needed the space, there were so many people. I thought Kaz was going to die."

I detect a new sound in the environment: a slight hiss. A malfunctioning monitor? One of the ceiling speakers?

"And then, twenty-eight minutes after the seizure started, it just stopped."

Yes. A hiss. But was it always there? Am I just noticing it now?

"Everyone cheered, then they all went away."

I pick up my chair and move next to her. With my hand resting on her knee, possibilities play out in my head: Kaz doesn't make it to the CT scanner because he seizes on the way, he's rushed back to the emergency department; or, Kaz makes it to the scanner but he seizes inside the chamber, he's rushed back to the emergency department, the aborted scan means that the scan will happen again, nearly doubling Kaz's dose of radiation; or, the CT is done but the scanner shows white-blotch-within-grey-blotch, hallmark sign of an intraparenchymal brain bleed; or, the scanner shows mass effect, the dense black hole of tumour; or, he could get a scan and the results are normal, sweet blessed normal—that being what I want, I think about it the least; or, I go crazy doing this.

Janet has something worse on her mind. "Will he be the same when he wakes up? Will he still be able to talk? Will he be able to grow normally?"

I've never been normal. In the time it takes me to answer, I believe yes, but then my belief wavers and I regroup. In another instance of medical logic paralleling relationship logic, I recruit belief. Reassurance is the key principle of doctoring. "I think he—"

Janet cuts me off. "Will he get to be in love with anyone?"

A BENT POPPY AFFIXED TO HER POCKET, Zee's little voice is raised for a poem by John McCrae about fallen men from long ago. She leads the elementary school choir, singing "In Flanders fields the poppies blow" before other students gamely join the tune.

In Guelph, McCrae's birthplace, specifically the auditorium of Victory Public School, we stand in a brick structure built shortly after the conclusion of the First World War. This place. Made in that time. To celebrate. The choir kicks in:

> The larks, still bravely singing, fly
> Scarce heard amid the guns below.
>
> We are the Dead. Short days ago
> We lived, felt dawn, saw sunset glow,

I am wrenched into a strange daydream. In my mind, the choir is drowned out by a host of fallen men, some headless, some missing limbs, who enter the auditorium hopping and crawling. Some climb to the rafters, one swings from the basketball net, and the remainder sit in empty chairs. Swelling the song, they too take up the tune, sing:

Loved and were loved, and now we lie
In Flanders fields.

The men's bodies testify to battlefields, whizz-bangs, and poppies. Blood begins to extend from the ceiling like thick spit. Is a flower the right metaphor for war and death, even one that's blood-coloured? After Zee's schoolmates sing *To you we throw the torch*, the fallen men respond in baritone, *Be yours to hold it high*. The song, almost done.

If ye break faith with us who die
We shall not sleep, though poppies grow
In Flanders fields.

I am, of course, flagrantly unwell. Who else sees and hears such things as these young children sing?

Are men defined by their sacrifice, by the loss of what they loved, by what they saved? Stop. Think of something else. There are other poems. There are poems written by Zee. Think of them. Those poems are her without me, her free of me.

Snow

Snow is falling from the sky covering our
ground with a thick white blanket.
Saying good night to flowers, grass and leaves.
We go to the store and get new mittens hats and snow pants.
It is a wonderful time to play outside, to
make snow men and have snowball fights.
It is almost Christmas time and we are
counting down the days with a
homemade advent calendar.

I love the snow times

GOOD ROUTINES PREVENT DISTRESS and obviate the need for soothing. I wake up in the morning at the same time. I go to bed at the same time. I start work at the same time. I eat at the same times. I develop a schedule to match my circadian biology and the interaction reduces the requirement for a different kind of soothing, a trickier kind: on-demand soothing. This kind requires either an activity to self-soothe, or another person who can help.

As a child, I was never taught how to self-soothe. There were rarely other people who could help. A few days after I had my first seizure, Scott, a young blond boy, tried to pull my ear from my head. "You talk too much," he said. "I'm tired of listening to you. Since you hurt my ears, I'm taking yours."

We all need soothing and will continue to need it. When Kaz is angry and unhinged, in seek and destroy mode, I say, "Duck Story! Let's do Duck Story!" And miraculously, Kaz will stop mid-smash, walk over to me at the laptop, climb up on my lap, and say "Ba dum ba dum."

I'll click on a link to a YouTube by Forrestfire99 called "The Duck Song" and we'll watch a music video about a duck annoying a man at a lemonade stand. Kaz and I notice the man get progressively angrier, his crudely-drawn face adding extra hilarity as it transitions from happy to enraged. "Man mad!" Kaz laughs. "Man mad mad mad!"

When the YouTube's over, Kaz and I roam the main level of the house while singing the tune, soothed.

A LITTLE-KID-COLONY CLAMBERS over a play structure moored on an island of crushed rock rimmed by black plastic. Should the kids fall from its moderate height, the shifting rock softens their impact. Boys compete to dangle from the bars. Girls prefer to sit underneath the plastic stairs and slides, talking. On the side of the playground adjacent to Powell Street, a boy jumps rope with a small group of girls. The only girl playing wall-ball is an expert head shot artist. The boys run in fear of the sniper when they make a mistake. A safety-jacketed teacher supervises the island, sometimes smiling when a boy's been picked off. Where is Zee?

In the southwest corner of the playground, a group of boys shout, jump, and point as part of a chaotic variant of soccer baseball that involves both throwing and kicking. A mid-sized boy launches the ball into the air, striking a baserunner in the head; the runner falls, screaming, and the group slowly approaches the fallen boy, now crying and holding his left eye. In a second, he's up—it was all a feint! Having lured them out of position, he races along the base paths, still holding the eye. So not a complete feint. As he crosses the painted home plate, the boy thrusts his non-eye-holding arm up in the air. Victory!

Adjacent, another game unfolds: girls in a chalk-demarcated square lob a ball with varying force at changing angles. Each girl must remain in her assigned area; the ball must land somewhere within her zone. The girls stand on the fronts of their feet, not fooled when the thrower looks up at a tree. If a ball bounces out of bounds, the failed receiver is replaced with another girl waiting to play.

Roving groups of boys throw baseballs and footballs to one another, making the playground look like it is constantly bombarded by projectiles. When these boys get too close to the smaller kids that swarm over the play structure, the teacher tells them to move back. Older girls stand in small groups to talk and laugh. A mix of other boys and girls play indecipherable games: perhaps hide and seek, kick the can, a chase game, touch football.

But where is Zee? Is she out there somewhere? I can't see her. I watch from the second-floor window of my house across from Victory Public, waiting for my daughter to appear. Is she on the other side of the school, hidden from view? After twenty minutes, the bell rings and children go back inside. Little kids line up at their door, the teacher sorting them according to class; big kids stream through their separate door in no arrangement or order. The teacher is the last to enter, her flock successfully recalled.

Victory Public has several windows facing our street. Zee's fifth-grade classroom is one of the classes whose windows face me, but those windows are too reflective to see through. If only it were midnight, if only a cat tripped the sensor, I could see inside. But then Zee would be here. I should remember to check on her then, to confirm that she is here.

THE SLEDGEHAMMER

I am seven years old. My mother stands on our stoop, a clutch of flyers in her hands. She reaches deeper into the black mailbox and pulls out a brown cardboard box with my name on it. I take the small package to my room and close the door. Inside the box, a holy rosary shines from the overhead light. Countless times I've seen old women in church pews bending forward, rosaries hanging from their necks, the crucifix clutched in their hands.

What is forgiveness, except of sins? I put the beads around my neck. After supper, installed in front of the television, I finger the beads as B.A. Baracus pities the fool. Just before bedtime, my father arrives home, his boots leave wide-stance mud tromps on the carpet. He booms, "Supper, woman!" Then he looks at me, swaying.

"The *fuck's* around your neck? You a faggot? You get those in your mother's drawer?"

"No, Daddy. I got the beads in the mail. They came in a box."

"Get them the fuck off." He lurches forward, overturning the coffee table on his way. He rips the rosary from my neck and shakes the beads in my mother's face. "This what you do, woman? This what you do, make my son a faggot? He wears necklaces and plays dress-up?"

"It's for prayer, Doug."

"It's for homos. Gaylords and sexuals. For shitdicks."

By day, Dad wears suits to work as a civil servant. By night, he drives a Massey-Ferguson tractor to sell topsoil from his dead father's fields. To work in this way is to have a mind divided. To work this hard is unnatural, unsustainable. And: he is not Catholic, has never held a rosary before. Why isn't it burning his hands?

"Fool outta me. Fool outta me. Fool. Outta. Me." He pulls a pint of Captain Morgan from his right pants pocket, drains it, and then throws the plastic bottle at my mother's face. Then he decamps into the bathroom with the beads. My father loves to be clean and loves telling me that if I feel sick, the best thing I can do is take a shower, just like him. "Wash the fever away boy. You can't get better unless you're clean." He is often ill. This is the most frequent piece of fatherly advice he gives. The pipes feeding the shower kick and hum for a long time.

I hide in my room, for the signs of the domestic apocalypse have come nigh. Through my bedroom door, I hear my father roar out of the bath. "Come see the god pile, Liz. Lo, the Lord has come unto our shithole tonight, sweet jaisus, praise glory be."

I hear the sounds of dragging underneath long screams. The trajectory of the screams moves from the living room to directly across from my bedroom. I stand from my bed and look out the window. But I'm not looking, I'm thinking—the pastime. Was this the first instance I had a conversation with my friend, Burning Crown Jesus? Until then, I'd often seen him just looking at me, mostly smiling, and rarely crying. He never spoke.

This time, Burning Crown Jesus speaks, his tongue more blood-coloured than the orange flames from his crown. "You know that I will always be here for you," he says, so calmly, so lovingly.

He's an adult, so I don't know what I'm supposed to say back. Am I supposed to talk to a window? So I don't. Instead, I think: *Yes. I know.* I'm not sure I agree with what he said. But I don't want to contradict. This was Jesus I was dealing with here.

The screams stop. I hear my mother moan, "I'm not cleaning that up." Then: a beating. A dull thump, closed fist hitting a back; steps, then a stomp and another scream. A brutal order. She says, "No."

EVERY SUNDAY MORNING, I went to church with my mother. Some Sundays, my father didn't come home the night before. Other Sundays, he was sleeping off a drunk. On the rarest of Sundays, he was awake on the couch, smoking, watching us leave. "Going to save the world, praise Jaisus?"

I always found this very funny, one of the moments we could truly connect. "I am going to get saved!" I would shout, pumping my fist. "Hallelujah!" Looking back, I expect this routine hurt my mother.

"Don't say a prayer for me," he'd always respond. "I'm too far gone. I'm goin' to hell! AND I LOVE IT."

"Ha ha ha, sinner! I'll be up in the sky, and you'll be deep in the ground where it's melty hot! Ha ha ha."

Everyone knows that true salvation requires praying for the lost. Perhaps this is what my mother was thinking, for she never said anything during these exchanges. She stayed with him until she died. Perhaps she prayed for his deliverance the whole time, but the best God could do was keep the possibility alive.

A YEAR AFTER HE FELL FROM ATOP THE TRUCK, I'm driving with my father along the Saint John River. As we cross the Burton Bridge on a fall day that features the mildly agitated water flanked by sponging willows, yellow birches, and red maples, he says at the midpoint, "Throw my ashes into the Saint John." I have heard him say this a thousand times since childhood, and always in the same place. Winter. Spring. Summer. And, of course, fall.

We wind along Route 2, the old Trans-Canada highway, until we reach the former site of our farm, sold just a few months before to pay the bills that accrued due to my father's accident. A re-possessor drives our red Massey-Ferguson tractor onto a trailer that is clearly too small. City fool. Halfway up, the Massey tips over and falls on its side. The re-possessor leaps from the seat, narrowly avoiding being crushed. Once down, the large back tire continues to spin, revolving the tractor until it is now pushing against the trailer.

I find this farce incredibly funny—another case of a city boy not knowing what to do. My father, though, says nothing. Either he remains invested in something that was once his, wanting the best for his past equipment, or he's genuinely concerned about the fate of the twit who just almost killed himself. It's hard to know. When did he ever care about anyone except himself? He treated that tractor like absolute shit, pushing it far too hard, day and night.

He breaks his silence only when we pass back over the bridge again, as per the ritual. But this time he says something I've never heard before. "I'm sorry," he says. "I'm sorry I treated you so bad." Tears fall freely down his face.

FOUR WEEKS INTO MY FATHER'S COMA at St. Michael's, my brother, sister, and I are still taking bedsit shifts. Doug's chart sits at the foot of the bed on a combination dais/desk. Jay, Doug's nurse, looks up from his perch after entering a note and says, "I hope you become a good doctor. It seems like you care."

Jay's cool. He tells me about the kind of medical resident I should never be, how the nurses will get back at me if I'm a dick. He teaches me about power paging: a resident will feel the wrath of a unit's worth of nurses who will slow-ration tasks all through a long call night if that resident is unpleasant to nursing staff. "Don't be a dick, Shane."

"I won't, Jay. I promise."

Jay seems satisfied with this. He goes to do the turn-and-wash on the neighbouring patient, an "MCA stroker with a huge hyperdense sign who never shoulda been tubed." Or so I hear some of the nurses say at the station. "When he stopped breathing, Doc Jackass did a resuscitation," Jay says. "As fucking usual."

Slosh slosh and fft ffffft goes the sound of Jay's gentle brushing from beyond the next curtain. Jay is entitled to instruct me in care, to interrogate whether I really give a shit, because he is a People Who Care. He tends to my father not as meat but as a person. He complains about things, sure, but who doesn't?

Slosh slosh. Fft ffffft.

Laughter sparks from the far corner of the unit and dies. Then movement—my father's right index finger, spasming to life. It claws up from the deep, furrowing the blue blanket covering his legs.

"Jay, Jay, Jay—his finger's moving! It's moving. It MOVED."

The finger stops moving. The adjacent curtain pulls back slightly. "It's not moving," Jay says, only his face visible.

"It did move, Jay—I saw it. Really." Do I want the old man to come alive? I do. I care for strange, inexplicable reasons. Not People Who Care reasons. Oh no. Mystical ones, praying-for-the-lost kind.

"This happens sometimes, Shane. You know that. You must have seen some families want a sign of consciousness so badly that they interpret involuntary motion as a sign. Tell you what. I'll back down on the sedatives and check your father's GCS in a bit to see if you're right. Okay?"

Jay cares. But this time, he cares coercively, relying upon co-membership in the medical fraternity to sell his rationale. Jay gives me a pitying look and then his head disappears. He resumes washing the MCA stroker, a man whose name I don't know and never will. He's more than a stroker, though. He's like my father. Unlike my father, he has no son to sit by his bedside. At least, not a present one. Maybe a ghost.

Slosh slosh. Fft ffffffft.

I will Doug's right index to move again. My thoughts extend in a laser beam to the index as an animating force.

Slosh slosh. Fft ffffffft. Slosh slosh. Ffffffft.

The finger moves again, contracts and extends; Doug's eyes open, and his head begins to shake slightly and twist. He coughs, triggering the pressure alarm on the ventilator. This means that Jay doesn't need me to cry wolf. The curtain pulls back again, and Jay's head and I both witness my father's face turn towards me. Doug's index finger slowly rises with his hand towards the ceiling.

My father is. Pointing. To. The. Ceiling. He cannot speak because of the tracheostomy, but he coughs because he's nevertheless trying to talk. He looks right at me while pointing straight up.

Boy. There. Get the sledge. It's right in front of your goddamned face.

But there is no sledgehammer here.

DOUG REPEATS THE CIRCULAR ARM MOTION many times over the next few days with increasing violence—and always looking at me, only doing it when I'm around. Jay puts my father in feeble wrist restraints, tying him to the bedrails. The care team's afraid he'll rip out the tube.

What finally makes me understand is reflecting on his *wrong, slow, stupid, on-purpose, asshole* wavelength. Pointing to the ceiling means he's impatient, as usual. He doesn't want to wait for anything. For no one. Especially not me. Doug points at the ceiling *because* he can't talk. After all, air flows through the tube, unable to make it to the larynx. My father points at the ceiling to say, *I want to get the fuck out of here, asshole. Get me out of here. Right. Fucking. Now.* But the natural response of the care team to his desire is to place him in restraints.

BCJ POINTS AT THE CEILING. "Lord my god, why hast thou forsaken me?"

Pharisees rush to the Christ and bind his arms and legs, rendering him unable to punctuate any further complaints with gestures. BCJ can no longer hide out in the garden of Gethsemane to gather his thoughts, to reflect on the nature of the drugs the Pharisees slip into his water, trying to get him to recant his teachings, to renounce his godhood, to disband the cult of Jesus. The Pharisees found his hideout and this is a raid. Jesus messed with their shit and fucked with their supply.

They will take BCJ to Golgotha, place of a hundred thousand dead bodies, where they will kill him. My own personal J is going to die, will sleep in the sand dunes with the rock hyraxes. I must save him. I must remove him from his bondage, prevent his eventual scaffolding. I must get him out of here, take him to the Land O Gulps, and perform the transubstantiation. The fate of the world depends on it.

OPEN UP
YOUR HEART

Once upon a time there was a little girl named Zee. She was smart and inquisitive, and she said "Hmmmmph" whenever her parents told her No, or Maybe, or Wait. When they asked why she said "Hmmmmph" when asked a question, she responded: "*I* say 'Hmmmmph' 'cause *you* say 'Hmmmmph.'"

Zee, are you going to zip up your bookbag? "Hmmmmph." Zee, did you remember to lock the door? "Hmmmph." Zee, I love you! "Hmmmph."

"Daddy, will you take me to Big Park?" Hmmmmph. "Daddy, will you make Rice Krispies with me?" Hmmmmph. "Daddy, will you colour with me?" Hmmmmph.

WHILE KAZ GOES BACK AND FORTH TO HOSPITAL, Zee complains of abdominal pain. Mental checklist of the most common physical causes of recurrent abdominal pain for a pre-teen child: heartburn; lactose intolerance; constipation; urinary tract infection. Less common causes: Crohn's disease. Intestinal obstruction. The most difficult cause of all, because there is 'nothing' to find: functional abdominal pain. Zebra cause: envenomation from the black widow spider.

"Dr. Yellow's office," said a voice that seemed displeased by the existence of life elsewhere in the universe. "How can we help you?"

It is more than possible for a health care worker to ask how they can assist while also conveying that they really have no desire to help; indeed, that the prospect of help is like a carrot suspended by a stick, held in front of an ass. The greatest amongst such negatively skilled practitioners suggest, in their intransigence, that help itself is impossible, so why expect it from anyone? Such an attitude rises miasmically from the ground up, from porters and sanitation engineers, and it pours down from administrators motivated only by two forces: cost-containment and complaints. Those caught in the middle—People Who Care—move through this universe of bland obstructionist villains.

I try to convert Mad Receptionist Voice into Mollified Receptionist Voice. "Hi. I'd like to book—an appointment! For my daughter, Zee. She's got abdominal pain." This is delicate work. I am cracking a safe with a stethoscope. I am calculating the number of raindrops that fall in one square kilometre as my body hits the ground at 9.8 m/s^2. I am juggling a chainsaw as I sing "That's Amore," Dean Martin-style. I perform the ritual abasement ceremony, key to be seen on the same day: "I'm sorry to be calling. I know how busy the office is. People calling all the time!"

Carrot. Gimme carrot. Gimme, gimme carrot. Me want carrot. Me a hungry ass who needs carrot. I achieve the slight tonal shift from very pissed to quite harried. "How long has she had it?" Mollified Receptionist asks.

Carrot closer now, yummy carrot. Need. "About a month I think."

"Then it's not acute," she snaps, back to sharp gatekeeper intonation. Oooohhh no. Gained ground lost. I gave the wrong answer. Evil Receptionist of the Distant Appointment gives me a faraway time. She is not a People Who Care. Carrot snatched back.

But she's right, isn't she?

The malignant causes on the differential are Wilm's tumour, hepatocellular carcinoma, neuroblastoma, lymphoma.

Hmmmmph.

ONCE UPON A TIME there was a little girl named Zee. Like her mother, she was crafty with her hands and built intricate objects. Popsicle stick dollhouses, toilet paper tube dragon snouts, cardboard ring worms, pipe cleaner spiders—Zee often led other children during craft exercises, functioning more as teaching assistant than learner.

One day, she brought home to her father a paper clip bent into the shape of an angel. The contorted metal was fastened to a cloth band. The little girl named Zee wrapped the band around her father's right arm and said, "Never take this off. This angel is for you." The father said, "I promise." The angel fell off, but the father kept it safe in his wallet, and uses it as an alternative rosary. On some days the father can be found muttering *BE OK BE OK BE OK* as he rubs the pink paperclip between thumb and forefinger.

WHEN WE EVENTUALLY SEE HIM, Dr. Yellow asks Zee the same questions I asked weeks before. Her answers don't point to a specific cause. Then Yellow presses Zee's tummy, causing her to grimace. The pain seems to be everywhere.

There is no window in Yellow's examining room, of course, but there is a computer screen. In its inviting blackness, I hallucinate Zee at three years old. I tickle her sides until, grimacing, she screams, "NO TICKLE!" The sides of the monitor begin to turn opaque, as if a fire was approaching from all sides.

Dr. Yellow does exactly what I would do. He orders a urinalysis and culture, a flat plate x-ray, and an abdominal/pelvic ultrasound. Zee disappears into the bathroom to fill the bottle, listening to the nurse's instructions on the way. "Just read the words on the door if you forget what I say, honey!"

Yellow looks down at his feet with Zee out of the room and says, "Is there anything happening at home?"

"Like what?" I ask.

Yellow's office is under construction. A cacophony of saw, drill, hammer, wall shake, and ping. Ping. A new noise to add: the pull of polyester on cotton as Yellow's white coat moves over his shirt—a very loud shoulder shrug. What are the actual building materials of new health care structures and renos these days? Bags of not-help and pallets of uncare?

"Kaz has been in and out of the hospital," I say. "It's probably epilepsy—"

Zee returns. There is something beautiful and wrong about a little girl holding a full urine sample bottle. Yellow says, "Good, Zee, we'll test that and do other tests that won't hurt at all. No needles! Then we'll see you and your dad back here." Zee smiles, holding her belly, slightly bent forward.

Walking out of the clinic, I'm confronted by the worst window of them all, the bright blue sky overhead. Brilliant sun, no cloud cover; my thoughts go there to die, to burn. Sky as place where I made a binding contract, *Don't let my son die.* But rather than suck up all my thoughts, this time the sky sends a thought down to me: *Shane, the age when you were first ill was nine.* The sky resumes its usual unidirectional gravitational pull, hoovering thought into itself.

Roaring upward: *No. Not that.*

ONCE UPON A TIME there was a little girl and her name was Zee. Zee's fifth-grade teacher called her father one evening, something that had never happened before. Was Zee in trouble? Was Zee bad? "I just wanted to tell you something remarkable, something really special," the teacher said. "Today at recess there was a little boy being bullied. A group of kids led by Zee's best friend were following a boy around and throwing things at him, including rocks. But Zee had the courage to stand up to them and protect the boy. She took the boy to one of the playground monitors and asked them to take care of him."

"Wow," the father said. "That's so good of Zee."

"What I'm really proud of is that she didn't just go along with the other kids even though it was her best friend who led the group. That really showed character."

The father didn't mention to the teacher that he had never been shown this kind of care when he was a child. What he did say: "I will take this very good Zee for ice cream tonight."

Zee, already: a People Who Care.

ZEE'S HANDS MOVE OVER HER STOMACH. She looks like she's in pain— face tight, lips turned down. "Zee, are you okay?"

iCarly plays on our one television. Carly Shay and Sam Puckett host a DIY web show. Carly, the tall lead, admonishes shorter, scarier Sam about her volcanic, titanic, frightening, cavemannish anger. Sam just blew up at Freddy the tech guy for a minor glitch that wasn't Freddy's fault.

Carly and Sam are never pictured with parents. Without parents, the social laws that govern the show make for fantastical possibility. As a pre-teen, Carly is responsible, genuine, and caring—even though she's apparently facing one of the greatest traumas children can face, living without her mother and father.

Carly, it seems, is made from sugar and spice and everything nice, a doll come to life. And for her part, Sam seems better off without her mother—an offstage presence who is only mentioned in the context of punchlines involving abuse. Being parentless is reinforced as a good when you consider the two main adults on the cast: Carly's older brother Spencer, who acts as Carly's nominal guardian, is an irresponsible twit who only gets in touch with his inner adult when the show needs that to further the plot; and Freddy's mom is an overprotective monstrosity, a needy nag who embarrasses Freddy in public.

"Yes," she answers, pain instantly vanishing from her face. I wasn't supposed to see. She concentrates on the show. Gentle, beautiful Carly coaxes Freddy to talk to brutish, also-beautiful Sam again. "You know her," Carly says. "She's *Sam*. She can't help it."

Zee turns to me, a blank look on her face. Her expression doesn't change as she stands and heads to her room upstairs.

Hmmmmph.

Janet's at work, completing her residency. My vision of a perfect television show: on *iParent*, a mommy and a daddy take care of a daughter harmoniously, with difficulties resolved by conversation, and respect shown by all family members to one another. By the end of each episode's twenty-two-minute run time, whatever hilarious conflict presented itself would be tidily resolved: a cooler *Full House*.

I'm by myself here. And if I'm the only one, then maybe Zee is parentless after all.

ONCE UPON A TIME there was a little girl and her name was Zee. Her father was telling her a story but he was only telling her a story in his dream. So, there was a little girl, and her name was Zee, and the father was telling her a story; but it all happened while he was asleep.

The father stared out the window for hours. Three symmetric slivers glow, mounting to an intensifying orange. A second or two later, the radiance dimmed. Ascending Exhibition Street, a platoon of ambulances hurtled into the emergency dark—five of them. The father lost track of how long he sat in his upstairs bedroom, alone, contemplating the change of light in the schoolyard outside. Somehow he fell asleep on the bed still thinking he was awake, looking out the window.

He remembered that he forgot to tuck Zee in with a bedtime story. How could he have forgotten? He stood and walked down the hallway to Zee's room, a wall-mounted nightlight weakly throwing blue to an opposite wall. Zee's room was pitch, but a blocky shadow could be made out on the uppermost shelf of her room—the butterfly habitat.

The father listened carefully to Zee's breathing to determine if she was sleeping. He heard slight whimpers, as if she were having a bad dream, so he gently sat down on the edge of her bed and stroked her hair. "There there, little girl named Zee. Everything is okay. Everything is okay, little girl named Zee."

But when he finished speaking, the little girl named Zee screamed. The father jumped up and turned on the overhead light. On top of Zee's tummy, a spider made of shiny black pipe cleaners slowly lifted up and down. Before the father could catch or kill it, the spider walked off the bed, climbed the wall, and sat back down on the uppermost shelf, near the butterfly habitat, where it had been for years.

AT THE END OF NOVEMBER, investigations come back negative, yet the mysterious abdominal pain persists. Hmmmmph.

Zee's fifth-grade class works though a poetry unit, tackling a new form each day. Zee spends her evenings perfecting haiku, revising acrostics, relineating free verse, restarting sonnets, reciting limericks. Above all, she's concerned about whether her lines are ready. In one of three piles of discards on the kitchen table, the uppermost poem lists over forty breeds of horse, each of these existing in a different setting: a field, a stall, a track, a park. The only shared elements are that the rider is a little girl named Zee, and on every page is a central depiction of horse and rider. The images look joyless, the horses a simulacrum of a dream. Dull brown of dirt and hide. The sky, black. The grass, yellow.

Another discard focuses on snow, its short text decorated with blue-outlined flakes. This snow poem is written in grey ink, formally deployed as a dense block on the page. When I started writing poetry, poems with wide-set shoulders were my preferred arrangement too. Better to carry the weight of the world, the mass of thought.

When a poem of hers is finally finished, Zee reads it aloud to me. "This one's Done, Daddy. Is it a Good Poem?" she asks, speaking in capitals-mode. As she reads, I can almost agree that the whole world is, yes, horses horses horses! Almost.

Her work during poetry unit borders on the obsessive; she makes small change after small change, mimicking how I write, but there's a joylessness to the drive. "What do you think of *Open Up Your Heart* as a title for my poetry book, Daddy?"

The kitchen window accepts the offering of my thoughts:

The name of my first book of poems is Exterminate My Heart. Whoosh to window.

This has nothing to do with me. I need to save her. Whoosh to window. *No.* Whoosh to window.

Stop pathologizing the experience of this little girl. Whoosh to window. *She's not you.* Whoosh to window.

"It's a great title, Zee. I think everyone should try to live up to it."

Expressionless, Zee says "Good," and, whoosh, returns to her room.

As early as 5 AM, I often find her downstairs, already at work on her poems. At night, if I wake to use the bathroom, she's sometimes sitting up in bed with the light on, still scribbling out words or redrafting stanzas. Having devoted my life to poetry, I understand the need. I tell myself she'll get bored by it.

ONCE UPON A TIME, there was a little girl named Zee. Her father told his psychiatrist about Zee's pain, and the doctor—Dr. Pink, named after the girl's favourite colour—asked a very simple question in response: "What do you do when your daughter is scared or sad?"

The little girl named Zee's father had no idea. He honestly didn't know; who teaches such things? Who was there for him when he was scared and sad? The father needed specifics, a more fleshed-out situation. Did Dr. Pink mean if there was a bully at school, or one-of-the-little-girl-named-Zee's friends were moving away?

"No," Dr. Pink said. "This is important. You don't need a fuller picture. You just see a sad or scared little girl. What do you do?"

The father didn't know.

"You spend time with her."

ZEE WEARS A PRETTY CANDY-STRIPE DRESS. In an hour, Janet will take her to a friend's birthday party in Stratford—little Ena's, blond child of an oppressively harmonious household. The party is in a dance studio. Hide-and-seek, cake, and salsa lessons promised on a colourful invitation festooned with rainbow unicorns.

"Do you think I'll need dance shoes?" Zee asks.

"Dance shoes ... like tap shoes?" I ask.

"Bring sneakers," Janet advises. "The instructor will get you barefoot anyway."

"I want to do my nails, Mommy," Zee says. "To be pretty. All my friends have their moms do their nails."

"Okay but not your toes," Janet says. "Toes are a waste if you're dancing."

"But if I don't have shoes on then everyone will see my ugly feet! And that's the *perfect time* for pretty nails," Zee whines, "when people can see! Everyone knows that!" She stomps off to clinch the argument.

But she has to come back if she wants to go to the party. When she does, she sits in front of me, looking as if the bottle of green nail polish she holds in her hand is intended for some other little girl in some other, better life. "You don't love me," she accuses.

Window-ward, I think: *but I've never loved anyone more before.* Whoosh.

I don't say it, the window took it. "Let's not be late for the party, Zee. You don't want to miss the Macarena."

For a moment, even Zee's favourite silly dance can't make her move. But then it does.

ONCE UPON A TIME there was a little girl and her name was Zee. The little girl stopped getting invited to birthday parties. She brought home her lunches untouched. She didn't read in the evenings anymore. She wanted to go to sleep long before her bedtime. She lived in her room like a refugee, only coming out to use the toilet. One day, her father asked her to come to Big Park with him. "No," said Zee through her closed bedroom door. "I am not a Park Person anymore. I do not want to go with you to parks."

The father said, "But if you don't come with me to Big Park, then who will I play with?"

"Hmmmmph," said the little girl named Zee. The door stayed closed.

The father said, "I will be sooooo aloooooone," drawing out the *o* sound as if he were a howling, sad dog.

"Hmmmmph," said the little girl named Zee. But movement could be heard behind the door, so the father waited. After a few minutes, the door opened a crack. "I will come to the park with you and be a Boring Park Person on one condition."

"Anything," said the sad and lonely father.

"You must get me a horse and we can keep it in our backyard. Horses are not boring." Since this is only a story, the father agreed, and the little girl named Zee and her father played in the park until Mommy called them home for supper, a meal the little girl didn't touch, soon returning to her room and closing her door, only coming out again when the horse arrived the next day from Horses "R" Us.

ON DECEMBER 21, the last day of the school year, Zee looks drained. *Open Up Your Heart* is due and she is sure the poems aren't ready. "The poems suck," she tells me. "They're no good. I tried and tried but they're just no good." Outside, snowmen built by schoolchildren stand as sentinels along Powell Street. They inspect the first pedestrians of the morning. Zee should join them soon—she is scheduled for crossing guard duty and has been late to report to her post many times this month.

"Zee, you've got to hurry!" I say to her as she rifles through a sheaf of poems in her hand, still crossing out words.

"But the poems aren't *readddddddy*."

Everyone has had to adjust to Kaz's illness. We're all sad. But then some of us experience sadness as an illness, one that wrenches our perceptions and leaves us unavailable to others. Did I lose track of Zee's sadness, so much like my own?

In my personal and professional experience, depression is not a siren. Instead, it's a soundless receding, a disappearing act, an unrevealing. And then, sometimes, yes. Sirens.

A few minutes later, on my way to work, I drive past an on-duty Zee at the corner of Powell and Exhibition. She wears the yellow and orange caution vest all the patrol kids must. Even though I slow down, hoping to catch her eye, she doesn't recognize me, just waves me on like any other car.

When I arrive home that evening, she's in bed. I sing through her door, "Zee, come and see me! Zee, you are my Baby Zee! Why be sleepy when you can be with me, the Daddy!" She refuses to come out, though, even though it's suppertime. "Food, Zee. Food is saying, 'Come and eat me. I, Food, am Yummy.'"

Before I go to bed that night, I knock on her bedroom door once more. I ask, "What did the Madamester say about *Open Up Your Heart*, Zee?" Madamester is Zee's kerchief-wearing grade five teacher.

I hear Zee's muffled voice, some sniffling. "She said 'Good.' But she said that to everybody."

"Did Madamester see how much work you did?"

"Hmmmmph. I guess."

"What else did Madamester say, Zee?"

"She liked it. I TOLD you. Mmmmph Daddy, I'm SLEEPING."

That midnight, I stand in my kitchen, watching snow through the old window. It falls fat and wet, sticky enough to adhere to the glass. Zee slowly descends the stairs. I know it's her without seeing because she has a quiet, orderly gait. She holds a book in her hand.

"I want to give you this now, Daddy. It's your Christmas present."

Open Up Your Heart is laminated and spiral bound. On the cover, a crooked, snow-coloured heart is encased in a red box. The kids must have been making these books for their parents all along, the deadline a way to force them to get the completed product in on time before a final book-binding trip to Staples.

I open it, happy to have something that Zee has made. Poetic repetition comes through serial representations of horses and a little brown-haired girl whose name is Zee. The poems are beautiful, alive, do not suck.

"I really wanted you to have it," she says. "Because I won't be here." With a resigned smile on her face, Zee walks past me with another copy of the book in her hand. "Mommy, I've got another copy of my book. I want you to have one too. To remember me by."

Do this, in memory of me.

I look to the window, hoping for BCJ to come. Please come.

No—I need not to fracture, not fragment; I need to stay here, not walk down the trauma hall and pick a different door. Stay here. Help.

Zee looks down at the floor. Then I notice. She's been crying. The current smile is more recent than the tears. Crying for how long? "I don't want to be here anymore," she says. "I want to die."

"Oh Zee, oh no, oh my god." I grab hold of her, *Open Up Your Heart* still in my hand. "Oh my lord." I cannot stem a torrent of thought whooshing towards the window: *This is a love story this is a love story I need this to be a love story.* Only now does Burning Crown Jesus appear, though faintly, in the window. An adult version wearing the golden crown holds a swaddled baby version of him wearing a smaller crown. The larger Jesus's flames slowly trickle down to the baby's crown, doubling its radiance. A flame transplantation.

THE DEVIL'S SWILL

Somehow, it's morning again. Janet appears over my face, blotting out the ceiling. While folding a shirt, she bends down to kiss my forehead. "Early morning for me, even though it was a late night!" Kaz can be heard synchronizing an unfolding series of crash disasters. Boom. "Do you want me to get him dressed this morning?" Whack. "It's the least I can do, since I have to go and might not be home until tonight. I'll be doing the EEG tomorrow, though. My turn." Whomp.

In these, the early days of Kaz's illness, we thought we could manage both our professional responsibilities and share care of him. It seemed simple: take turns either going to work or going to hospital appointments. At some point, though, in the face of a serious illness, a choice is forced on a family. It comes sooner or later, but it comes. And then you look in the face of your partner and you wonder what your marriage is made of. From his room down the hall, I hear him holler a serial refusal to put on a diaper; to wear clothes; to brush teeth; to move.

THE HOSPITAL BAG IS PRACTICAL. Unlike a satchel of amazements one might wish to take to the other side after death, to heaven— containing things like a lucky coin, a pink angel paperclip, a tinfoil halo—the bag must be brought when Kaz goes to the hospital, and it must contain useful things. Diapers—so many. Board books. Blocks. Two sippy cups, red and turquoise, perhaps for lemonade or the devil's swill, who knows? Three changes of clothes. Trickiest of all, one must leave enough space for Harambe, the only stuffy who matters, Kaz's sleep toy god.

"HE WAS SO GOOD!" Janet reports. We sit in the den, the night dense outside. "Even the tech said he was easy. But funny story: at the end, she placed an electrode in Kaz's hand and said, 'Kaz, this magic button reads your mind.' Kaz looked amazed and said, 'Magic?' After considering it for a few seconds, he tried to eat it but when I told him no, he stuck the electrode to Harambe's head and pretended he was conducting a magic show. Shane, he actually told Harambe to fall asleep, just like we told Kaz to! But Harambe doesn't sleep. He jumps up and down on the bed instead, and continues jumping all the way out of the hospital, off walls and desks, as Kaz chants ''hrams NOT sleepy mommy.'"

I MUST CARE FOR KAZ as BCJ cares for me, always there, always on call, ready to save the day, and actually saving the day, except I can save nothing, I cannot even save myself. In this way, the circular logic dictates: BCJ will need to save both of us, adding to his burdens, but then BCJ is a figure for everyone, meant to save us all, who has saved us all already.

But Kaz is still seizing. Kaz has not stopped. Who have I ever saved? Is there any saving anyone, anything? Can I take the relief that Kaz has stopped seizing with me when I go?

A month ago, Janet and I agreed to share responsibilities, covering for each other when it comes to career obligations. Janet had a shift in the necropsy lab? I was on duty. I had an evening shift at work, the only time some patients can see their family doctor? She was on duty. Appointments with the pediatrician, our family doctor, a phalanx of phlebotomists—all, in theory, to be equally divided.

The unspoken issue between us is that Janet put her career on hold for a couple of years while I completed a family medicine residency. Delaying *her* residency isn't fair. The other disruptive force in our marriage is my mental illness. Experiencing terrible sleep, a deluge of thought that leaves me adrift on its own tide, muttering about the sky, but never disclosing the fact of BCJ, his reality—the uncertainty around Kaz's health is killing me.

I'm in a double bind. Taking a parental leave from work would allow Kaz's illness to become my focus as opposed to a distraction. The time off would also function as sick leave, hypothetically allowing for my own recovery. The problem with this thinking is the nature of my despair itself. Kaz's illness is necessitating the ubiquity of BCJ, his omnipresence, my constant need.

Janet turns on the television using the remote. An American serial about a high school glee club pushes sexuality as close as possible to the censor's line. Without turning towards her, focusing instead on the window, I say, "I'm not sure we can keep up with Kaz's care the way we're doing things now."

No response.

"Do you think that one of us needs to be the main caregiver for Kaz, so that things are better organized for him? We've already missed a couple of appointments over confusion about who was supposed to do what."

A musical number. Why do they increase the volume on these? Still no response. "Janet, are you listening?"

"What do you want to do?" she non-answers, eyes not budging from the program. A beautiful someone jumps over someone else; now the group forms a pyramid. Isn't this a glee club, not a cheerleading club?

I could say that I'm getting sicker, that I'm overwhelmed, that I don't know what to do. I can never say that BCJ is in the room beside us, watching the program, titillated by several of his comely works. But I think that she knows the first part, and what would be the point?

Nothing is resolved in this conversation. The show is obsessed with sex and pregnancy; half the young women are having sex, and everyone's talking about a disgraced pregnant girl, something something immaculate conception. Classic teenage shame plot. In a moment or two, my gaze is back to standard window mode, unspeaking, waxy flexibility.

The next morning, I request a leave of absence from work.

KAZ'S MEDICINE NEEDS TIME TO WORK, but I need his medicine to start working in the same way my father needed instant gratification, pointing in the air with his index finger and making short circles as if he is creating a tornado in the sky. *RIGHT NOW RIGHT NOW RIGHT FUCKING NOW.*

The monitor hisses into my right ear from its perch on the window ledge. Napping at the moment in his bedroom, Kaz could seize anytime. Seizures don't care where he is, or when. Seizures are like my father. They come when they want, they do what they want. They have all the power in the world.

THE PHONE RINGS. "Hello, is Dr. Neilson there?" The voice sounds silky, young.

"Yes. Speaking."

"I'm Dr. Cerulean, the pediatric neurologist." Why am I being addressed *by* a physician responsible for the care of my child *as* a physician? Then I realize: the referral to the neurologist must have mentioned that I'm a doctor. "I have the results of the EEG."

When a doctor calls immediately after a test, the result is never good. "Okay," I respond.

"Your son has independent spike foci in the left central and right occipital areas. As you know, this means that there at least two places in his brain that are causing his seizures. The test doesn't say *why* these areas are there, just that they are present. The areas declared themselves when Kaz started falling asleep and when he started to wake up."

This detail about awakening isn't surprising—spike wave patterns are more common in liminal states. More surprising is that Dr. Cerulean's news is worse than expected. *Two places. Two. Not just one,* I think. *Two places means the seizures are harder to stop.* A Seuss-inspired snippet springs into my brain:

> *Bad Spot 1 says, "Your turn to make him drop."*
> *"O thank you, Bad Spot 2. But really, after you."*

"I should see Kazoo soon," Dr. Cerulean says.

What if Kaz seized? *What if he needed someone to save him? To care? We're bonded now, he and I. We've got to get out of this together.* The kitchen window seems unsatisfied with this collection of thoughts. It glimmers for another one. Hit me, it says, gimme another. *Maybe there is no saving me if I don't go somewhere else, do something else.* The window stops moving in light, seems more restful. Sated. Satisfied.

IN CHRISTIANITY, epileptics have a bifurcated fate. If lucky, they will be considered to be saints, especially if they work as priests or monks. If unlucky, they are deemed possessed by demons and evil spirits. The Bible's one crystal clear case of epilepsy is described alternately in Mark 9:14–29, Matthew 17:14–21, and Luke 9:37–42. A young boy is brought to Jesus: *And one of the multitude answered and said, Master, I have brought unto thee my son, which hath a dumb spirit; And wheresoever he taketh him, he teareth him: and he foameth, and gnasheth with his teeth, and pineth away.* Jesus commands the man to bring forth the boy, who is said to seize as soon as Jesus lays eyes on him: *straightway the spirit tare him; and he fell on the ground, and wallowed foaming.* Jesus asks how long the possession has been present, and the father responds that the affliction has endured the entirety of childhood. What happens next is desperately sought by me, indeed is the project of my belief. Jesus declares, *If thou canst believe, all things are possible to him that believeth.* He then commands the spirit to leave, but the spirit causes the boy to have one final seizure as it exits, producing a fit so potent that many gathered at the scene thought him dead. But Jesus takes his hand and the boy rises, cured.

Kaz rises after each seizure, not cured, and with each new seizure, cure seems less possible because I believe a little less, resurrection a familiar miracle: with each seizure, the boy is struck down, stilled, and yet the boy rises again. When he makes it as far as he can, for as long as he can, he falls. Then a mother and father take care of him. Worry about him.

I HATE PEDIATRIC HOSPITALS more than any other kind. The McMaster Children's Hospital comfortably occupies a middling status amongst that garish group. A mishmash of brutalist concrete and brick exterior, with a parking lot so ridiculously tiny that a team of men must guide parents into spots that come due on the clock, its interior trying and failing to be welcoming to kids in the same way the parking lot fails and the exterior fails. As in, each component of the hospital is barely useful. Looking at the structure, one wonders why both beauty and utility have been abandoned as a principle.

Walking the main floor, one notices how the occasional brightly coloured clinic exterior fails to blend with the overhead mass fluorescent lighting and vinyl tile. Same goes for the spiral wishing well, the coin-operated Rube Goldberg machine, and the hospital foundation auction display for a mounted AC/DC album. Look more closely and you'll see that the wishing well's coin spout is plugged with gum; you're warned away from the Rube Goldberg machine with an out-of-order sign; and no one wants the AC/DC memorabilia, for a notice says the item's been held back for two months so that a bid might come that recoups its cost.

Perhaps I am being unfair. Maybe all the beauty to be had from hospitals can be decanted from wisdom brewed in the emergency department: there is no beauty except the kind you bring in, so hold onto it for dear life.

The 2G clinic is an oppressive yellow, the same tint as the crayon children use to make the sun. The pediatric neurologist is slim, a few years younger than me. His voice seems higher in person than it did on the phone, but still silky. "Hello, Kazoo. You look like you need toys. Do you need toys?"

"Kaz-WHOAH" Janet says, as if it matters. "But we use the short form Kaz."

Kaz takes in the strange new man who entered the room who speaks such magical words. *Toys?* his expression says. He's not sure.

Kaz has a two-second assessment time if you are Good for Him or Bad for Him, akin to my adjudication of People Who Care status. Kaz is intuitive and predictive, whereas I am deliberative, assessing evidence after the fact. It is always harder to know what Janet is thinking.

Consider Thomas the Apostle, his hands hovering over Christ's wounds. Seeing is believing for people of little faith, but the concept goes both ways. Christ understood this point supremely well. So much of medicine is selling yourself so that your advice is received. The additional factor of parents—their wariness and concern—makes an awareness of marketing even more important.

Noticing the colourful trunk in the man's hand, Kaz seeks further confirmation. "Dere toys dere?"

Why do I hate hospitals so much? There is my own personal experience, of course. When one has to live in them as an involuntary patient, one comes to develop a certain distaste that isn't necessarily the fault of the hospital. The other reason is simple professional exposure. When I was a young medical student and resident, I smirked at the old people's perception that hospitals were places you went to die. Where else are people supposed to go to be cured? Over the years, I learned that they are completely, utterly right. These places were designed to deal with death in bulk.

The doctor says, "My name is Dr. Cerulean, I do have toys you will play with and like very much. I have lots and lots of toys." He sets down a dented and scuffed red box.

Where did he get this routine, *The Cat in the Hat*? Will Thing 1 and Thing 2 jump out? Will the doctor don a red-and-white-striped top hat and say, "Your mother will not mind at all if you do?"

I turn to Janet, but as usual, there's no telling what she's thinking. I'm leaning perilously close to *not* a People Who Care.

Addressing us as dyad, but in the plural, he asks, "Parents? How are you?" Though the phrasing is technically a question, he says it flatly, like a statement. He sits down and opens his laptop, but when he notices that Kaz has not yet investigated the colourful trunk, he lapses back into singsong. "Kazoo, go ahead. See what's inside!"

"Actually," I remind him again, "his name is Kazuo. We call him Kaz."

Dr. Cerulean smiles at this information, but still doesn't say Kaz's name. Instead, he opens the trunk himself and pulls out a purple bouncy ball. "See? Toys!"

There are several levels of medical bribery available to physicians. The first, and most basic, is the promise of stickers or a lollipop when the visit's over—*if you're good*. Stickers for those who prefer—kids like options—but also for the parents who don't want their child sugared up. The second, technically more assistive and facilitating than a true reward, is demonstrating how medical implements work in the examining room. If there is an otoscope, show the child the magic trick of transilluminating your finger, then their finger. Point out the electronic switches that raise and lower the level of the bed and let them whirr away for a few minutes. The third and ultimate level is toys. Toys are serious. Toys mean medical business. Children behave for the promise of toys.

Cerulean has an unfamiliar use for toys, one reserved, I suppose, for specialist pediatricians who must take long histories from parents. He uses toys to buy time to take the history again, beginning with the story of SNAAARRRKKKKLLLLK.

A purple ball hits me in the head.

We progress to more recent emergency visits and admissions. Kaz finds a small die-cast ambulance that is a perfect replica of Hamilton Paramedic Services buses. The ambulance smashes into the purple ball. Ball gets its revenge by bouncing into the ambulance, toppling it.

As we talk, Cerulean fills in an electronic questionnaire, staring at the screen as he runs down his checklist. I begin to worry. No toybox is bottomless.

Kaz finds a plastic sports car that revs when reversed, storing potential energy, and screams forward when let go. Cerulean has to speak louder due to the noise. But he picked the toys.

Kaz finds a plush orange rubber reflex hammer. In my mind, he becomes Medical Thor, god of lightning. In a sense, he is a little deity of electricity—struck from above like a bolt from the blue, then coursing on the ground with energy conducted into his body. Leaving Janet to answer Cerulean's questions, I point to my knee. "Kaz, whack here. See my reflex." Kaz whacks the ambulance instead, then the sports car.

He finds a wooden shape puzzle. "What dis?" he asks, shoving the puzzle frame towards me from the floor. "Puzzle," I answer, dumping out the shapes and placing a robin shape back in its nest. Kaz is uninterested in restoring the puzzle to its previous state. Instead, the shapes are more fun to kick.

Occasionally, Cerulean glances at Kaz as Janet and I answer questions. This means he's doing triple duty, compressing time as much as he can: taking a history, writing notes, and examining the child.

Janet asks, "Do you think there's a way to stop these seizures?"

"I'll answer any questions you have once the physical exam is completed and we've talked about the results of investigations," he says. Cerulean's permanent weak smile radiates no warmth, light or sense of home—just a soft-plastic professionality, a brittle armor against the world. Janet admits no sign of irritation or concern on her face. But I think I can tell, somewhere in her eyes, that she's beginning to distrust.

"Kaz, now I must play with the toys. I like toys too, you know. Let's share."

"Kay, I *very* sharey," Kaz nods, now completely liking this doctor with good toys.

Kaz hands Cerulean the orange hammer. "Sharey!" Kaz says, emphasizing the proof. Cerulean uses it to pretend-test Kaz's reflexes, tapping Kaz's patella and elbow as he sits on the floor.

"Trade?" Cerulean says, holding out the hammer while motioning for the purple ball in Kaz's hand.

"Share," Kaz says, making the exchange.

Cerulean moves the ball, tracking along an imaginary grid in front of Kaz's face. "See the ball, Kaz? Keep your eye on it! Don't let it get away!" Kaz tries to grab the ball, but Cerulean pulls it away to the extreme margins of Kaz's visual field.

"Me," Kaz says, stomping his foot. "My ball!"

Cerulean gives the ball back, mollifying Kaz. A few seconds later, Kaz throws the ball at Cerulean's open laptop, now resting on the examining table.

Cerulean pulls a fire truck from his pocket. "Doctor have toys dere?" Kaz asks, incredulously, as if the doctor were made of toys. Cerulean was holding out on Kaz, anticipating this very moment. He steps back slowly, nodding, encouraging Kaz to follow him, as if he were the pied piper, observing Kaz's gait, frowning slightly as Kaz chaotically toddles. What does the frown mean? It seems especially significant since Cerulean's default mode is permasmile.

"Kaz, what's over here?" the doctor says, looking to his left. Kaz follows his gaze, but the doctor's tricky, rubbing his right hand some distance from Kaz's left ear, opposite to the direction Kaz is looking.

Kaz is confused. Nothing is over there. Suspecting that Cerulean's hidden even more goodies, Kaz says, "Dere toys dere?" But on hearing the scratchy sound, he turns to the doctor's right hand.

"No fooling you, Kaz. No fooling you." He hands a stuffed monkey to Kaz from inside a drawer in the examining table. From Kaz's point of view, this room is amazing. Toys can appear at any time, from anywhere— the equivalent of magic. Kaz bashes the monkey against Janet's knee.

"Momma call doc-tor, doc-tor said," Kaz sings. We play this game at home, with Harambe.

Cerulean laughs, permasmile back in place. "Let me explain my thinking to this point," he says, focusing on Janet. "Kaz's diagnosis is epilepsy—but that word is nonspecific and has many causes. The CT scan from Guelph didn't show a tumour, but it's the brain as seen through foggy goggles. In that sense, CT is a lot of radiation for a poor look."

The verdict on People Who Care is about to be reached. The jury is about to be recalled to the courtroom. I think of the Cat in the Hat wearing goggles. He says: *I see the entire world this way, Sally and Henry. It's the only way the world can be seen!*

"Things can still be there that CT scans miss." Cerulean turns to me. I realize I hate him, I want the heat in me to melt his smile. "Dad, I've told you already that Kaz's EEG shows multifocal abnormal waveforms in the temporal and occipital regions. Do you both understand what I mean?"

I nod. Janet nods too. We researched the result online, using university databases. Cerulean points with his hands to the approximate place on his own head where Kaz's aberrant electrical activity occurs. Where would I point in my own head to locate the crazy? I'd mimic what the bullies did from my childhood, using my index on both hands to make circles around my ears.

"Based on Kaz's presentation and the family history you both share, I'd say it's either a genetic condition or random thing, most probably not a tumour."

Wait. Not a tumour, *most probably*? Smile smile smile, one big long stretch of smile. He thinks this is good news. Good, reassuring news.

Have I ever talked this way as a doctor—*your son could have something really, really bad, but most probably he doesn't?* What's the translation of such a statement into human? But then the art is not that the message is different in kind, for the same information has to be conveyed. The art is relaying the message in a way that recognizes how terrible the message is.

For some reason, a vision of the outside of the children's hospital comes into my mind. The compromise between cost and function sacrifices beauty. But what can parents do? This hospital has to suffice. There is no other, better place.

Something isn't right. The smile is constitutive but behind it is another piece of news, something not worth smiling about. "So Kaz needs an MRI then," I challenge.

"Yes, he does need one," Cerulean replies. "The question is when we can get it and if he needs it right away."

No, the question is one of beauty and truth. The hospital is ugly, the business done inside terrible, and the compromise struck between form and function is not the whole story of compromise. The other parts to the story are power and need.

I keep pressing. "Because it *could* be a tumour. Right?" This is a contest. To the winner goes the spoils. If I win, I get an MRI for my son. If Cerulean prevails, he holds back the demanding parental hordes.

"Yes, he does need an MRI, that's right," Cerulean says, as if a catch is about to be revealed. How can he remain pleasant at a time like this? The fake empathy displayed by my medical students during their clinical skills sessions would be better than this false cheerfulness. At least, in their case, the empathy remains hypothetical, an end-goal that may yet be achieved. Cerulean is where hope goes to die.

"Boing," Kaz says. "Boing boing."

"A tumour has to be ruled out. And this is the bad news, Mom and Dad." There is more bad news than that which we have already received? "Here in Hamilton your son will get an MRI in about twelve months. There's a real backlog, I'm afraid."

Kaz is to be sacrificed on the altar of resources and waiting? A previously healthy toddler with seizures needs an MRI as plainly as this building is plain. What if an unknown tumour grows and by the time it's identified, the cancer is inoperable? What if my son dies because of an entire year's delay?

Cerulean offers this explanation: "You see, the MRI is a sedated procedure. Kaz needs to be sleepy so he can't move, he has to be still." The doctor is not looking at us anymore. He's scrying in the laptop screen. Is this what it's like, talking to me as I look at windows?

"The equipment for sedation is plastic, not metal. It's special equipment. An anaesthetist puts him to sleep and watches him for all stages of the test. It's a big thing. We only do these kinds of MRIs in a block one morning a week due to our limited resources."

Cerulean's explanation is feeble, a flimsy defense for a pathetic system that can't care for a two-year-old with new-onset seizures. "But tumour *is* part of *your* differential?" I say, raising my voice. "Kaz has *focal* areas on the EEG that fit with tumour? And you're offering an MRI in a *year*?"

The doctor frowns—his smile is perturbable! "Well, it's not me that's *offering* the test. This is a *resource* issue. I can't justify ordering an MRI without focal signs."

Janet and I are being processed out. Sorry sir, sorry ma'am, this is just company policy. I would of course help you, I want to help you, see, but my hands are tied here, this is just the way it is. Yet we both know that if it were his son, or if it were his clinic's administrative assistant, boy howdy! There would be an opening this week. "Kaz has power in all his limbs, his physical exam is normal. The good news is that the CT scan didn't show anything... ."

First he calls the CT scan "a poor look" that isn't worth the radiation, as if it's unfortunate it got done at all. Next, we're told it misses things. And as the final part of the trick, the normal CT result is supposed to make Janet and me feel better? In the far-right corner of the room, Kaz flips the ambulance over and spins its wheels.

"... and without focal signs I can't justify the test to the radiologist."

Kaz shoves the ambulance as hard as he can. It decelerates as it crosses the room, eventually nudging the doctor's shoe. "I could make a referral to Sick Kids in Toronto. I could request for the MRI to happen there."

I suddenly, wildly love Toronto. Toronto is now a god I pray to. I take back everything I said about you, Toronto. Give my son an MRI and I will be yours forever. Cerulean's smile returns. "But in my experience, it takes nine months to get in. It's not a big advantage, timewise."

"Is dere toys dere?" Kaz says, perceiving he might go somewhere else now, some other hospital that might also have toys.

"What else can we do?" Janet asks in a calm tone. Why isn't she fighting too? Or maybe this is a good-parent-crazy-parent routine?

"I do have patients who can't wait and they go to Buffalo and pay for things themselves. I could do the referral today."

Can't wait? Fuck you. It's *won't* wait. "Yup, call the Americans," I say. "They can bail *us* out."

I have no idea what my face looks like. I never do. Inside, I'm a reactor, affect rising up and out as force. Cerulean looks at Janet, ceasing his engagement with me for the rest of the visit, choosing to work with the less emotional parent.

Kaz turns the toy trunk upside down, shakes it. Nothing's inside.

THE GOVERNMENT OF CANADA ratified the UN Convention on the Rights of the Child in 1991:

Article 1 defines what a child is. *My son is a child.*

Article 2 sets out the principle of non-discrimination: "[n]o child should be treated unfairly on any basis. Children should not be discriminated against based on their race, religion or abilities; what they think or say; the type of family they come from; where they live, what language they speak, what their parents do, what gender they identify with, what their culture is, whether they have a disability or whether they are rich or poor." *What good is a policy when my son can't get the investigation that he needs?*

Article 3 insists that the best interests of the child should be paramount: "This principle places the best interests of children as the primary concern in making decisions that may affect them. All adults, including those who are involved in making decisions related to budgets, policy and the law, should do what is best for children." *What compassion exists in a system that outsources care to America?*

Article 6 pertains to a right to life, survival and development: "Children have the right to live. Governments should ensure that children survive and develop in a healthy way." *My son could have a brain tumour, and my country is no guarantor.*

KAZ CRASHES THE AMBULANCE INTO MY BOOT. I tune back in as Cerulean continues to engage with Janet, the non-difficult parent: "... that last more than a half hour are potentially dangerous. This is called status epilepticus. At that point, the seizure should be made to stop with strong medication."

Janet asks, "Like what medication?"

Looking at his watch, Cerulean says, "You know what guys? My nurse Lemontine is very knowledgeable and she will answer all your questions. My job is just to take the history, do an exam, and then make recommendations."

Lo. Janet reacheth the Magic Question Limit. Cerulean's head pivots back to his laptop. Janet and I are expected to wait silently. Kaz crashes the ambulance into the wall. My hand tightens on Janet's knee.

A few minutes elapse. Finally, Cerulean stands and packs his toys back into the colourful trunk. "Bye Kazoo! It was nice meeting you!" Kaz hides the ambulance behind his back as Cerulean reaches for it, but then Kaz smiles and hands it over. "I sharey!" he explains.

Shortly after Cerulean leaves, Lemontine enters, her heels clicking against the 2G tile. Before retirement, my mother worked for over forty years as a nurse. She stood all day and developed pained, callused feet, her toes shoved laterally in hallux valgus. How can a nurse do heavy work in heels? How do they get to a medical emergency fast?

Lemontine hands Janet her card. "The doctor says you have questions?" she uptalks. Lemontine responds to most of Janet's questions by admitting she doesn't know the answers with more uptalk: "I'll ask the doctor later and get back to you?" We are trapped in a time-wasting buffer designed for Cerulean's convenience. Suddenly, insanely, I want the heat of my thought to melt Lemontine's heels down.

We leave the 2G clinic feeling hopeless. Kaz pushes the elevator button, Janet trying to guide his button-pushing madness towards the "P" that designates the underground lot.

Unlike brochures that feature pictures of orthopaedic success stories and cured cancer patients, hospitals actually emit a cursed energy. Just as we cross the threshold separating the elevator-protecting glass enclosure and the asphalt lot, Kaz collapses. I take off my jacket and place it under his head so that he doesn't get road rash. Janet turns him to the recovery position. People walk by—doctors, nurses, the fellow afflicted. Some are in a hurry and don't stop, staring at us as they wait for the elevator. A calm man puts a hand on my shoulder and asks, "Do you want me to call an ambulance?"

"No," I say, laughing, pointing insanely up, arm raised, index finger extended, making quick small-radius circular motions, just as my father once did. "We were just in there!"

Only a short seizure, one minute long. Kaz emerges from the underworld with his piercing keen. As his mother finally picks him up to her shoulder, he whispers in her ear, "Med-cine." The way ugliness works in this place is such that I will be sad to see the AC/DC display go.

KAZ SITS ON THE PIANO STOOL, straining to reach for the keys. *Go round and round.* He only plays a D syncopated to *The Wheels on the Bus.* For twenty minutes now, Kaz has risen back to life, but time is limited. He must seize again. In two minutes. Or in three. Exactly when is a mystery, but that he will is a certainty. *The wipers on the bus.* D, D, D, D, D. *Go D swish D swish D swish D.* I embody windshield wiperdom, swaying my body while waving my hands. *All D through D the D town D.* The rescue mat waits on the ground near the stool. If my son falls, I will catch him. When.

His head pitches forward into the keys, sounding a final D. As he jiggles, I lower him down to the mat and place him in the recovery position. White flakes stream past the window, some of the god-given stuff clinging to the glass, some already descending as melted streaks.

Mark the time.

Beach Boy Dennis Wilson, brother of Brian, faced a personal disaster in his life during the late 70s, forcing him to pray for salvation through song. Wilson fell on his knees in front of his piano, believing the song he needed was inside the instrument somewhere—he just needed to find it. Are pianos like snowflakes—no two sounding exactly the same?

Perhaps the piano is a god. It sits, quiet.

After three minutes and thirty-three seconds, slightly longer than it takes the duck to drive the lemonade man into a murderous, teeth-baring rage, Kaz returns. The first ten seconds, he silently gathers breath, about to emit the querulous homing signal to the world that I now call Lost Noise. For four hours more, the postictal effects linger, making him unsteady on the piano chair and slurry in speech. He cannot get clear, seizing again and again.

IN THE WINDOW, I conduct a thought experiment involving cartoon versions of God, Satan, and a common sinner. God is dressed in white robes, sporting a long white beard; an oily, florid Satan is moustachioed, with tail and pitchfork—the whole cliché. The sinner is a middle-aged father with a blank face and ill-fitting clothes. Both biblical powers set up competing lemonade stands on opposite sides of a busy road. God's brand is Yellow Acceptance of Any Outcome. Satan's swill is Medication Guaranteed or Your Money Back Brand (see Fine Print). The father inspects God's juice, then crosses the road to consider Satan's juice. Which should the father pick to cure his kids' ills?

Answer: he doesn't pick, because a large truck runs him over on the road.

THERE IS A POETRY TO MEDICATION NAMES, a strange concentration of generics that end in the suffix -ine. First generation: chlorpromazine, fluphenazine, perhenazine, thioridazine, thiothixene, trifluoperazine. Second generation: Olanzapine. Quetiapine, asenaprine, cariprazine, clozapine. On the wards, you can hear these drugs whine, the -ine boring into skulls, creating burr holes, dousing brains, putting out fire. In my brain. One to the next, try this and try that—my neuroatypicality mounting the resistance known as side effect, my body captured by muscular contraction. Acute dystonia: drug, drug, drug, clench, clench, clench. Take this pill, be clamped by vice grips.

Burning Crown Jesus is more than hallucination, delusion. BCJ is also defiance, a grandiosity with a brain that is beyond this world, that burns with literal holy fire. No one can put out that light, it burns eternally, no drug can tame it. *Impervious* fire. The *Oxford English Dictionary* defines the suffix *-ine* as "added to names of persons, animals, or material things, and to some other words, with the sense 'of' or 'pertaining to', 'of the nature of'." Pertaining to crazy, the nature of insanity, a song of myself that sounds like a laser beam, a space transmission from aliens, but which has nothing in common with the whoosh of Burning Crown Jesus's ecstatic inferno. Such is my fine drink, my sad discipline, that which knocks me supine, makes me bovine, that stalls my engine, that presses thought into a flatline.

CERULEAN MUST HAVE SENT THE REQUISITION the day we met, as promised, because a clerk in the radiology department of Buffalo Women and Children's Hospital calls me a day later.

"Kazoo is a girl's name or a boy's name?"

Over on the couch, anyone but me would think the soundly sleeping child beautiful, peaceful, but just thirty minutes ago he seized while drinking milk, adding the terror of choking and aspiration to my usual seizure drama. At the moment, Kaz rests in a middle stage, long after Lost Noise but still some minutes before rousing to drunken, uncoordinated activity.

"He's Kaz-WHOA. A boy," I say.

"We have the referral from your doctor." The voice is low, barely audible. "Says here you're from Canada? Then you should know the hospital fee for the test is $250. The radiologist charges $100 to read the MRI. And the anaesthetist costs more than that."

Perhaps the sound is so low because hope is so distant, and the conditions need to match? "How much?"

"Well, I don't speak for that department. But a lot more. It starts at $500, maybe, but the cost depends on how things go. They bill you when it's done. You can always ask them, of course."

What cheap lemonade. Being willing to pay ten times that price to get my son an MRI in Canada, a hundred times that much, a fridgeful, I ask, "So when can he get the test?"

"We do sedated MRIs three mornings a week. The soonest opening I have is ... let me check this again. Right. January 18, 11 AM."

A sedated MRI in less than a month? Kaz begins to rub his mouth, an early sign that he will soon wake up. "We'll take it." I speak as "we" now, for Kaz and I form a we. I'd put him on my shoulders and walk him to Buffalo if I had to. He and I would stop at all the lemonade stands on the way there.

On my laptop screen, Ernie and Bert fly across the sky in beds that trot like horses. The two friends arrive at a sky-city constituted of clouds while singing about a great adventure. Ernie and Bert don't sing of survival, but that's the kind of song I want to hear. Their song concludes on the word 'home,' that word held in one long, harmonious note. Kaz wakes as the single bed bearing Ernie and Bert hides behind a cloud. "'rahms," he murmurs. He wants his stuffy.

Out the window, elementary school kids from Victory Public threaten to vault the playground fence by heaping snow on the school side. The trick is to not quite make it all the way, to dangle a foot just a few centimetres from the ground, to pull back at the last second. Wag, wag, wag the leg. Watching them, I feel the luxurious naughtiness too. If anyone does make it all the way over, they must march back to the wide entrance archway where a woman wearing a caution vest metes out discipline. What she says, I don't know. But the offender is always banished inside.

Kaz seizes again, without his stuffy. I was too slow to move. I turn him on his side and see, in the window, that Burning Crown Jesus is watching over us again. He beckons me closer to the window.

I PRAY THE SEIZURE PRAYER: *please don't seize again.* Short seizure in the doorway. Short seizure on the couch. Short seizure on the stool at Brush Teeth Time. Short seizure in his bed. *Hiss.* Short seizure in my bed. Short seizure at the breakfast table with cereal in his mouth. Short seizure while playing with cars on the fireplace mantel. Short seizure trying potty. Short seizure after waking up from seizure.

Hiss.

Short seizure on my lap. Short seizure on my lap. Short seizure on my lap. There is no controlling the seizures, we are controlled by them. At this frequency, Kaz finds no daylight between seizure and consciousness. He either seizes or recovers in a postictal netherworld scored by Lost Noise.

Hiss.

Though valproic acid has been around for over 130 years, its antiepileptic properties have been known for less than half that time. A French chemist named Eymard first discovered the suppressive effect on rats while actually trying to prove something else. Spiritual journeys are much the same. Embark on a pilgrimage to find god, but know the self instead.

Most epileptics are controlled by the first anticonvulsant prescribed. After that, it can be a difficult trick to find the right drug or combination of drugs. Seizures beget seizures. By virtue of having a seizure, one is more likely to have another just because of a kindling process in the brain. Sticks rub together, then a forest fire.

THE GOLD INVITE ARRIVES IN THE MAIL, inlaid cursive—all class. "Please accept the invitation of Oprah Winfrey to participate in our Book Club this year. We would like to broaden the readership of *Saving* to a wider audience, because we feel that the book's core messages of love, care, and destigmatization should be shared. Oprah so loves your book—please see the enclosed handwritten message from the QUEEN."

"Dear Dr. NeilsOn,
  Your bOOk about recOvery and fatherhOOd is sO beautiful, I just must have yOu On the shOw. Brian WilsOn, Francis FOrd COppOla, Mariah Carey—as I'm sure yOu knOw, they have bipOlar disOrder. I've interviewed them all, such warm and lOvely peOple. If yOu accept this invitatiOn, I wOnder if they'd cOme tO the BOOk Club and chat with us abOut *Saving*'s message. We are gOOd friends, sO just say the wOrd, and I'll ask!
  Fingers crOssed you'll cOme,
  Big O"

The glossy insert of Big O, showing a standard headshot, reveals a face in perfect health. But scribbled into the white space above the photo in yellow crayon is a crown. Upon closer inspection, I see that O's teeth have been filled in yellow too.

A week later, at Harpo Studios in Chicago, Illinois, I'm sitting across from an irate Big O, challenging every single detail in *Saving*, demanding to know if I am truly as sick as I make myself out to be. There will be no Brian Wilson, Mariah Carey, or Francis Ford Coppola.

"Aren't yOu just impOsing yOur subjective belief upOn the reader?" Big O asks. "DOn't yOu wOrry a little bit abOut the sacrilege. I mean, 'pOwdered mOtOrbOat?" And all the misOgyny! Are yOu REALLY a dOctOr? Is that fake tOO? If yOu are a dOctor, why would they let crazy peOple intO the prOfessiOn?"

"Weren't you on the pipe back in the day, Big O? I know the show is big time now, fancy, sponsored up to the heavens. But it wasn't always this way, was it? You had shows with strippers and drag queens just like the other daytimers."

Big O has been doing this a long time. She's boxed with the best guests. "YOu want me tO turn my fact checkers lOOse On yOur ass?"

If cancel culture has taught me anything, it's TRIPLE FUDGE down. I mimic flicking a lighter, holding it steady over an invisible stem, and inhaling, humming "I Got So High That I Saw Jesus" all the while. I mean, c'mon. Big O my ass. This is the big JC we got in front of us here, the hOliest of hOlies.

Big O fires one final shot. She's skeptical of how few MRIs there are in Canada. "That's a lie, Shane. That's a lie."

"But Big O," I say. "You've seen all this yourself, with your own eyes. You see all and know all. You know what I say is true. You are the Queen of all Media, ruling even the divine airwaves."

"MOre denials." Burning Crown Oprah turns to the audience and says, "FOr example. MRIs are nOt hard to get. LOOk under yOur seat, audience, and get yOurself One free MRI, Of any part Of the bOdy yOu want!" A huge scanner is wheeled in from backstage, instantly sucking the change from everyone's pockets. "We'll dO it nOw! Mehmet Oz, my Peter, lent us this frOm COlumbia University Medical Centre. Let's see if y'all gOt tumOurs! And remember all yOu watching Out there: create the highest, grandest visiOn pOssible fOr yOur life because yOu becOme what yOu believe. Okay, let's cut tO cOmmercial."

WHAT AM I SUPPOSED TO DO FOR HIM but wait? In time, Kaz gradually wakes, groggy and wobbly, slurring. Though he shouldn't walk, he's incapable of comprehending should and shouldn't. Only two years old, all uncontrollable id, he pulls himself up to walk only to pitch forward or backward into a wall or table end. I hold both his hands to move him around the house as if we are dancers at a bar, one of us having had too much to drink.

Over the next few hours, I prevent major head injuries. Round and round the room we go, toys here, toys there. Kaz parks cars around the edge of the coffee table until he drops, convulsing again, just three hours after lorazepam flakes ghosted his lips white.

More useless prayers for the little sacrificial boy. *Please do not seize again. Please do not last. Please stop. Stop stop stop.* When the latest one's done, I buckle Kaz in the car seat and make the pilgrimage to Hamilton, the cabin light on in case he turns blue.

SOME DAYS I WAKE, not knowing how long I have been asleep, sun pouring in the window. Afternoon, morning, it makes no difference—Janet has to cover for me, or not. Is Kaz sleeping too? Did Janet put him to bed? Is she even here? On other days, I cannot fall asleep and so stare out the window all night, pouring thoughts out.

On one of those days, who knows exactly when it was, I walked down the upstairs hall to find that Kaz wasn't in his room. Or was it one of those nights? Perhaps I was asleep, reliving the jump from a height, falling a centimetre a minute in slow dream-time, or reliving one of Kaz's seizures, so familiar, the monitor's hiss summoning me: *save him*. But I keep walking past his room and scale the water tower, each rung up an increasing release.

I feel something in the window now, something good, and pull back a bit to get focus. BCJ's here, in the sliver of orange light. He's crying again, which according to our implicit understanding, means Something Bad Is About to Happen. His tears flow down towards a set of wire cutters. There are bad things BCJ can't, or won't, stop from happening, and I really appreciate the early warning system. I can brace myself. He says, "By a name, I know not how to tell thee who I am. Had I it written, I would tear the word."

That same day, which could have been any day, which was most days, the first part of the nightmare features the bedroom window. My conscious experience starts and ends with windows. I look at Victory Public School, stolid against the sky, blocking the view of the north part of the city. The school's Canadian flag flaps in the wind. The light outside suggests oncoming evening. Or brilliant morning. Or night. What time is it, exactly? I think: this is like a different life. Where am I? Did I die? And then I take the steps that end with my death.

Before I start on the journey, though, I always see a woman in a puffy brown coat pulling a boy in a short red sled. Why didn't I notice before? It's snowing. Was it snowing before? Or did the snow just start to fall? The boy wears a black snowsuit. I don't know why these details matter, maybe they don't matter. The woman and the boy move east, towards Exhibition Park. As they cross the street in front of my house, the boy loses his scarf in the wind. After a few skips, it halts mid-street on black ice. The woman continues on, unaware, but the boy turns around to watch the scarf leave him.

I need to stand to see them continue to move. They travel further into the park, passing the ball field, stopping for a moment at the outdoor skating rink. Perhaps the boy notified his mother of the lost scarf. Or maybe they are making plans to return to skate later in the day. The scarf remains in the street, whitening in the snowfall. When I look back at the rink, the pair are gone. The scarf gradually disappears, buried under snow, and when I detach from the window, it's dark outside.

Am I dead? This feels like a different life. No—not dead. I must go to check on Kaz. No, the water tower. How many times has my son's head struck the snow in the past two winter months? If this isn't a nightmare, then have I really slept for the whole day? I dress and go outside to retrieve the scarf. No. I'm walking to the water tower.

IN MEDICINE, SLEEP IS A SO-CALLED "vegetative" symptom of mental illness in which one can either have too little, or too much. In the *OED*, the first definition of the word has it that, "In certain philosophical and theological systems: designating the soul, or that part of the soul, which is associated with the most basic functions of life (growth, development, reproduction) as distinguished from sensation and reason; having such a soul." The medical view is largely in line with the *OED*'s, but the obvious disjuncture comes with "soul." Biomedicine is all sensation and reason, quantification, the accumulation of data, and it says nothing about the quality of life, about subjectivity. Biomedicine has no soul.

We abandoned crosses, sweeping archways, and stained glass for bland wards and crowded rooms with an overhead television spewing out the twenty-four-hour news cycle. We exchanged beauty and made a strange surrender for an illusion of control, and while doing so we gladly gave up our souls. Because biomedicine is the dominant player, the *OED* admits the definition of "vegetative" is "Now chiefly *hist*," meaning historical, out of use. We secularized it, gave it to medicine or medicine took it from us, who can know what the new gods do? Now the term is understood as

"7.b: Chiefly *Medicine*. Characterized by visceral functions only; having autonomic nervous function only; *esp.* lacking consciousness, cognitive function, and voluntary movement."

Think of a farmer, hoeing cabbages all day, long rows. Or perhaps sowing mustard seed, and tending the plants, ensuring adequate amounts of water and fertilizer. He chooses the terrain wisely, rich soil, and closes out the summer with a bountiful crop—enough to sell, enough to enter the winter season when the lights go down, when there is more darkness, when there is snow, when—ironically—it is likelier that vegetative symptoms might take hold. In this winter, the farmer stares out his window, or perhaps he is merely captivated by the window. He sees Burning Crown Jesus in the glass, hoeing cabbages while drinking a Diet Coke, humming *Even better than the real thing.* Or his vision penetrates the glass and he tries to calculate, in a single instant, the number of snowflakes falling in the scene. Lo. The number cannot be counted. He pulls his vision back to the window, its shimmer, and sees Burning Crown Jesus atop a red Massey-Ferguson, wearing a straw hat, hayseed in his mouth, hands off the wheel, arms spread open wide, staring directly at the farmer, shouting: *If I should count them, they are more in number than the sand: when I awake, I am still with thee.*

THE EMERGENCY LOT'S SMALL, much smaller than one would expect for a hospital this size. A short line of cars fills the front row. Kaz didn't seize on the drive. I prayed to the god of seizures the whole way. A fickle god. A capricious god. He smiled on us off-stage. No BCJ accompanied us in the windows.

BE OK BE OK BE OK.

A long, makeshift tunnel made of plywood and orange tarp leads to the interior, making for an exhausting walk carrying Kaz's postictal dead weight. Over and over again, this sign reappears: THE EMERGENCY DEPARTMENT IS UNDER CONSTRUCTION. But who wouldn't get the idea?

Once inside, I approach the desk clerk protected behind a glass window thick enough to be bulletproof. The desk clerk bleats, "Health Card?" I hand her the green plastic with the Trillium on the front. "Reason for visit?" she bleats again.

Trash Heap has spoken. Meaaaah.

"My son makes Lost Noise," I say.

BE OK BE OK BE OK.

The clerk pulls back slightly from the glass, shaking her head. I am broken? I am broken. I have lost my mind. "Seizures," I say, mimicking her head motion, stifling the urge to wave my arms as if mimicking the action of flame.

Kaz is slightly more aware. His head slowly swivels, taking in the room. "Toys," he slurs.

"All right. Have a seat and the nurse will be with you."

Meaaaah.

I recall the sign of peace from St. Vincent de Paul long ago. Fellow parishioners turned around in the pews to shake hands with men and women ahead and behind, saying *Peace be with you.* And at the conclusion of mass, the faithful are released by the priest when he intones, *Peace be with you.* The flock responds, *And also with you.*

Kaz has had fifteen seizures today. Rather than be satisfied with the holy politeness take-your-indifferent-shit-from-reception protocol, I say, "My son's had *fifteen* seizures today." I point at a large splotch of vomit in the centre of the room. "You should get him seen now because he's going to seize on that floor."

"Sir. You have to wait. There's a lot of emergencies today. We're really backed up." This is her sign of peace, her responsorial. She might say it a hundred times a day. A janitor approaches the splotch with mop and pail. The only thing to do is wait, but waiting makes no difference. At a glance, I can see that Kaz is the sickest person in this emergency department. Every other kid—all five of them—are awake and alert.

The most important thing any doctor can learn is not diagnosis nor prognosis nor therapeutics, but instead: be able to tell when someone needs saving. Forsooth: I perform the act of prophecy. "You're going to let him hit number sixteen and only *then* will he be put to the front of the line. Nurses and doctors will rush into the waiting room to put him on a stretcher. Let us past the gates."

The clerk isn't impressed, now leaning towards the glass. "Please sit down *sir* and *wait*, the triage nurse *will* see you soon."

I lift up one of Kaz's hands to the ceiling and then let it go. "The nurse will see *him* on the ground, convulsing. I hope *you* see him too. I hope *you* are the one to get the nurse to come."

"Sleepy, is he?" she says, turning her gaze to a set of papers on her desk.

Concerns around infection militate against toys in the waiting room. While I sit, I try to time each *BE OK* to Kaz's respiration, holding his arms to prevent him from falling unprotected onto the hard floor.

BE OK BE OK BE OK.

At the twentieth breath, Kaz seizes, the prophecy foretold. Why call out? Why say anything at all? I kneel beside my son, putting my jacket under his head, close to where the vomit splotch used to be. Another father, alarmed, runs to the clerk, gesticulating at the child on the ground. The useless cavalry comes, and I'm too exhausted now to look at the clerk to make an "I told you so" face. I've got other, more pressingly useless things to do—a new round of waiting.

There's some shadow in the clerk's glass, something familiar in the corner of my eye.

"BURNING CROWN JESUS, why can only I see you?"

"No one sees anything, Shane, other than what's really there."

"But people look right at you, Burning Crown Jesus. You're really there. And they don't see you."

"I am really here, Shane, but I'm here for you."

"I thought you were here for everyone, Burning Crown Jesus." BCJ's flames rise a little higher and seem a little more sinuous. I need to stay in my station and know my place.

"I know you love your son, Shane."

"The love does no good, BCJ. It does no good. I am only with him; I can do nothing for him."

Burning Crown Jesus moves closer to the hospital plexiglass, blackening it. "It is with love that I remind you, Shane. *Fear thou not; for I am with thee: be not dismayed; for I am thy God: I will strengthen thee; yea, I will help thee; yea, I will uphold thee with the right hand of my righteousness.* Do you believe that being with another is the most powerful act?"

And so I say it, the sacrilege. "I believe in the water tower." With a sudden hiss, the flames are doused and BCJ is gone. Shocker: I have the power to snuff out the light.

MY BLANK, MOONLIT FACE stares out the bedroom window at water tower, water tower, water tower until Janet enters the room. "Do you want to go to my concert?" Janet asks, her long black hair meeting between her breasts. Janet plays clarinet for the Guelph Concert Band. Going to a concert seems as possible as taking to the sky, like superman. Except I don't want to be anywhere near the sky. If I'm close, it means I'm about to jump. "It's tomorrow," she adds.

Janet manages disasters by not staring at windows, stimming, or dreaming of a water tower. She moves through difficulty, ever pragmatic, maintaining self-care by continuing with the things she loves. She still meets with friends for coffee, whereas I have deleted my Facebook account. I open a laptop and see either Burning Crown Jesus or a mischievous duck on the screen, whereas she has a spreadsheet open, or is reserving hotel tickets, or paying credit card bills.

Small Guelph performances are usually conducted in churches like Harcourt United on Dean Street and the Unitarian Church on Harris; monster loud performances use the Sleeman Centre, home of the Storm Major Junior franchise, seating capacity 5,100; but the River Run Centre holds 785 comfortably, with an atmosphere like that of Toronto's Roy Thomson Hall, but better, because: smaller. Less overwhelming sensory stimulation.

I notice that Janet's brow is furrowed. Then I notice, too late, that I'm stimming *BE OK BE OK BE OK.* Trying to stop on demand just makes things worse—I need a regular rhythm to dispel the stim, something I can tie it to, to make it dissipate, but there is no such sound, so I generate one, tapping with my left foot.

"Maybe it's not a good idea. Kaz might seize," she says.

"No, I want to go," I said, foot tapping as if I'm impatient, but really, I'm trying to anchor myself to the world, not get sucked up into the sky.

I don't tell Janet the reason I want to take Kaz. She would think me worse than she already does. I believe that the music might do what the drugs can't—quell his disorder, stop the seizures. Soothe him. Expel the vibratory demon. There is a precedent. In the Old Testament, the treatment for Saul's suffering as caused by an evil spirit was King David's playing of the harp.

Think me foolish? Get reduced to your last chance. Believe you have nothing. Realize that your world is coming undone. Then tell me that magical thinking and delusions are a waste of time. Remember, all that there is to do is wait.

WE SHARE THE DULL BLUE ROOM with an adolescent girl who ineffectually attempted suicide several hours ago. She looks about fifteen and bears the stigmata of suicide on her face—it's the first detail I noticed. Residue surrounds her upper lip, all the way up to the philtrum, forming a black moustache. Some time in the immediate past, the medical staff administered charcoal.

A woman in a white coat enters the room, announcing herself as a medical student by the sheer volume of handbooks in the pockets of her coat, her body slightly slumped as she walks. She seems barely old enough to have completed an undergraduate degree.

Another helpful aid to distinguish between hospital doctors: the more senior the staff, the more like a regular person they look, the less encumbered they are. Knowledge and power hide within them as qualities. They don't wear knowledge like armor, having no ignorance to protect.

At first, the student is confused, staring at Kaz as if he is a problem. But then the student hears a groan from behind the adjacent curtain and immediately brightens. "Amanda?" the student says, still unsure.

The curtain doesn't answer.

"Amanda, I'm the medical student—I'm here to take your history."

At first, the curtain thinks it might avoid the student just by playing dead. But then it moans again.

"Okay Amanda, I hope you're decent? I'm coming behind the curtain now."

The life story of the young girl is very reluctantly told, with many sullen pauses and repetitive invocations of resentment and anger that are so familiar to me as both patient and doctor, formulations that always exist when one is despairing. One of the difficult truths of suicide is that there is a selfishness to the act, no matter how benignly the sufferer may frame it.

"Everyone hates me. All my friends hate me. And my family hates me. My mother and father have never cared about me, never. Everyone is so mean!"

The rendition is supremely ugly, but then so is my soul, right now, also hopeless. I just bear despair differently, by virtue of greater age. The teenager is just a few years older than Zee.

"I can see how that would be unfair," student says. "The doctors really need to know how much Tylenol you took," she adds, shifting the topic. The student has a one-two strategy: first, validate; second, gently move away from resentment and try to gain the necessary information.

Perhaps I underestimated this student. Her interviewing technique is advanced: by displacing the information requirement as if it is the imperative of someone else, the student reduces the resistance of the interviewee.

"Bottles," says the girl. "Whole bottles. Bottles and bottles."

"Why did you take them tonight, though?"

The curtain sulks out, "I don't know."

Though the girl clearly doesn't want to talk, the student keeps trying to extract her information in this switchless, fully lighted room. Kaz sleeps despite the glare. Do suicide attempts and seizure kids both need the spotlight? Will the new emergency department house toddlers and adolescents in different spaces?

Like everyone made to drink the charcoal, the teenager hated being made to do it. If left alone for a few hours longer, though, she would talk. Right now is too soon. She's angry with everything and everyone. But if the student gets the history now, before the staff physician goes off shift, she'll get a distinction, a good evaluation, extracting capital on the way to an exemplary career.

Kaz's nurse rolls in a trolley with a television, VCR, and cassettes. Children here can have their pick of dinged *Thomas the Tank Engine* and *Cat in the Hat* episodes. Maybe Kaz will wake up before seizure number seventeen. Maybe the infusion running into his arm will work. Which one of these shows would he like to watch? Perhaps the Thomas episode when that Very Useful Engine has a cold and cannot assist Sir Topham Hat's quest to vanquish the forces of Confusion and Delay.

But I cannot cue the show. Kaz seizes in the gurney.

COLIN CLARKE, A BLACK MAN WITH A COMEDIC KNACK, conducts. Janet plays second clarinet. She's wearing black pants and a black vest with a white chemise underneath. A painfully amateur emcee neuters the success of each song with cringeworthy introductory banter: "You know, if my mother could see me now, she'd say: you're doing such a bad job! But you guys don't care about my mother, right?"

Children carrying teddy bears take the stage. Larger children hold the smallest bears, and the smallest kids—as young as five—drag larger bears. The music strikes up and children make the bears dance.

Is this real? I'm beginning to doubt myself anywhere. The nightmare is gaining in its power, fooling me repeatedly, making me lose the things I love the most several times a day. Kaz, blue and dead. Zee, blue and dead. The children smile, wave bears overhead, then sit in a circle and pretend to picnic.

> See them gaily gad about
> They love to play and shout
> They never have any cares
> At six o'clock their Mummies and Daddies will
>   take them home to bed
> 'Cause they're tired little Teddy Bears

The tallest girl, perhaps ten years old, approaches the smallest boy. Her brown bear—nubby, well-loved, chewed by dogs—kisses his huge polar bear, something probably won from a midway stand. Janet's wet, streaked face blows into her clarinet. The children put their bears to sleep on their backs, arms and legs sticking into the sky.

Though nothing about this performance is beautiful, I have no need for beauty. Grief is looking upon a tawdry, uncoordinated performance involving children on a Guelph stage and projecting all the terrible hopes and pain one has for the future onto them, like a mirror of one's own life. The sicker a child gets, the more a children's song—any children's song, even the oppressive cheerfulness of *Cocomelon*—will break their parent's heart.

> If you go down in the woods today you better not go alone
> It's lovely down in the woods today but safer to stay at home

Safer at home? The band starts into "Soul Bossa Nova" while stuffed bears lie supine at the front of the stage. Colin says, "Ladies and Gentlemen, give a hand to the bears!" as a River Run employee sweeps the teddies into a pile and then pops them one by one into a black garbage bag.

MY SON ON THE GROUND IS A METAPHOR. That he moves purposelessly is a refinement of the same metaphor. He goes away and he might not come back—he's on a journey close to the earth. Sapped on a couch, with Kaz on my lap and "the Duck Song" playing on the computer screen, I ask myself: *will my son ever be free?*

Kaz yet lives with the strength to be sick and strut about the living room even though he could fall. After squishing play dough through an ice cream set, he approaches me with a toy stethoscope and says, "I doctor. Where you sick?" If any future patients looked close at Doctor Kaz, they'd see his precocity in the healing arts: he smiles at pleasing things, appearing very trustworthy.

I point to my head. He shoves the plastic bell against my eye. I go to a cupboard and hand him a real stethoscope. "Where I sick?" he asks. I point to his head. Thrilled, he takes the real bell and puts it on his nose.

THIS THOUGHT IS MOUNTING AND STRONG: *jump from a height jump from a height jump from a height.*

I get up and go outside at 2 AM. I think I'm going for a stroll, but just as so often in the nightmare, I've tricked myself. I'm actually walking to the Verney water tower, the very same temptation visible from my bedroom window. Like BCJ, the water tower is also there to watch over me, also something that knows. It is to caring what dysphoria is to euphoria, BCJ's opposite pole.

I arrive at the outer fence. I note the higher inner fence is made of much thicker wire. A ladder is the access point for city workers to scale the tower, but they'd need a ladder themselves to reach that ladder.

The next night, I wake again and go to the tower to confirm the details. And the next night. It seems fitting and calming to sit against the fence and pretend to know nothing, nothing at all.

When the Canadian Tire opens, I pick out the biggest heavy-duty wire cutters I can find. Then I load my light blue Aerostar van with an extendable ladder taken from the basement of our house. I am going to die. It is what I want.

KAZ SEIZES OFTEN ENOUGH that I've decided it's unsafe for him to sleep alone. After all, he could seize and I wouldn't know. I could wake up one morning to check on him and he could be dead. I might find him in the middle of a seizure and have no idea how long he'd been seizing, one minute or a hundred. So goes the catastrophic thinking aimed towards the window, Victory Public looming outside.

Kaz is a paradoxical creature, unable to fall asleep until he receives a long, wild rendition of "Wheels on the Bus" with ever-changing verses:

The chocolate bars on the bus eat the seats, eat the seats, eat the seats.
The aliens over the bus beam the bus away, the bus away, the bus away.
The sun melts the bus into orange goo, orange goo, orange goo.
The scary man on the bus plays loud music, plays loud music, plays loud music.

Every so often, I sneak a boring regular verse in. *Move back please, move back please.* "Scary man, scary man," he demands.

Janet climbs into bed at midnight, Kaz between us. Or at 1 AM. Or 2 AM.

NO FLOOR LIGHT BASKS THE OSTENTATIOUSLY CRUCIFIED son of God at Norfolk First Baptist Church. No candles are lit for the dead and dying in remembrance and intercession. This place spurns the Catholic traditions of my childhood. Perhaps because it is an echo of that childhood, I walked here instead of to the water tower. Perhaps Brownian motion brought me here, the probability of me as a particle (P) moving a quantifiable distance (x), and yet—here is the beautiful part—the total distance I have moved is greater than (x). The equation allows for linear and nonlinear distance alike.

In medical school, when my illness returned, we were made to sit in front of microscopes and regard microbes. Swab the mouth, rub saliva on the glass slide, put the plastic cover on top, insert onto the stage, look through the eyepiece, adjust the objective lenses, and then visualize bugs who have no tendency, who move according to no principle save chaos, microbes equally likely to move in any direction. Future motion was independent of past, and motion was perpetual, unceasing. The light shining up, I thought I saw evidence of god's work, his mysterious plan revealed. There is life, and it is random. Evidence of such at the macro level was not enough. A biomedical version of this evidence in an actual lab, as achieved through technology: rare demonstration of the mystery.

Despite the familiar high windows, soaring ceiling, pews packed too close for my knees, and red carpet running down the centre aisle, something's missing. Then I know what it is: Burning Crown Jesus, inextinguishable flames licking his hair. Time for a trip to ol' faithful: I look to the stained-glass window on my left. He's there!

"What can I do for you today, Shane?" Tranquil Jesus—a soothing version that amplifies the life impulse by the revivifying cast of his gentle light. Who knows, though, if he just slipped on those white robes. If, a minute before, he was Hef-ing it up, full grotto.

"Just you be you, Jesus. Don't get burned, and always be there."

"I will always be here for you, Shane. I know you know that."

"Yes, Jesus, I like that you know everything. It's very comforting. I don't know why I never ask you questions, though. I should. I might find some things out."

"What do you want to know, Shane?"

There is something I want to know, an explanation of the first divine mystery from the early days of my crazy. Was Einstein right in 1905 when he posited, based on a statistical mechanics approach, that the motion of a particle in a fluid was the product of the random difference between pressures around the particle? And are humans subject to such Brownian motion as they walk the earth, the pressure from above crushing their affects into depression, or an unbearable lightness creating mania?

Pretending not to hear, I don't ask. I want BCJ to be real, and testing him might prove him not to be. Besides, this knowledge might already exist, Googleable in the electronic Gaia. If the answer I might find during some keyboarding midnight of the soul differs from BCJ's, then doubt could become the daylight between Jesus's soothing words and my belief. And there can be no separation from the mystery, else there is no impediment or check, no break-glass-in-case-of-emergency option. S →↓.

Ahead of me in the pews, a little girl improvises melodies to words beamed by the PowerPoint projector. In a few minutes, she'll be summoned to the front for Children's Time. From there, she attends the generic Sunday School of a watered-down Christianity. So much more friendly, this church, so much more welcoming to children than the one from my childhood.

A woman in a wheelchair, moved by the spirit, throws her arms in the air, shouting, "Hey!" The stultifying air makes my legs stick to the pew. Then the woman shouts, "Praise be."

I look over to BCJ. His arms are in the air, and he shouts, "Hey!" too.

Like every Sunday, I lose track of the proceedings and think instead of other things. Random images—my little girl kissing a small snowman she calls her snowself on the mouth, breathing into her snowself's lungs, looking up at me wanting me to make snowself after snowself after snowself for her; my father in the haymow with his fists blocking out my vision. Memory flow according to Brownian motion, reminiscence particles thrown through doors that open because of microenvironment pressures in the cerebrospinal fluid. BCJ's looking at me now, his tear-streaked face reminiscent of the Station of the Cross where crucifixion nails enter his hands. That walk was not Brownian. That walk was foreordained, orderly, linear. "Shane, it's okay—you know I'm always here for you."

BCJ is both ethical and realistic. He doesn't say, "I can save you, Shane." He didn't when it mattered, when I was a child. But then again, maybe he did save me. What if he hadn't have appeared to me as a child? Was that how he saved me?

I know I'll never join the celebrations of these people. At least not like them, not like the woman and BCJ when they both throw their hands in the air, moved by the spirit to shout, "Hey!"

BCJ begins to disappear. He looks alarmed and scared. "I will always be here for you, Shane!" BCJ is my bro, my dude, my very own personal J. The little girl's singing—clear, high, and blissfully under the broad wing of a presumable God ↑—brings me back, either as cause or, perhaps, I returned because of Brownian motion, the equation for the action of God as follows:

$$P = \frac{e^{-x^2/4Dt}}{2\sqrt{\pi Dt}} \ .$$

ANOTHER SEIZURE CEASES. I lift Kaz to my lap as he reports from the Underworld. Lost Noise drops off after a few minutes. He suddenly flails his arms and legs in a tantrum burst. "I hate them too," I tell him. At the sound of my voice, he opens his eyes.

"I have YouTubes ready Kaz!" On the screen, the scene we've watched together hundreds of times unfolds again: a crudely drawn duck waddles to a lemonade stand. The duck wants grapes. Stand Man gets progressively angrier, his face evolving from friendly smile to grimace, then glare, and finally rage. But in the end, the duck and Stand Man become friends! Sort of. Kaz and I enjoy the homicidal truth in their relationship.

Kaz would laugh too, but he's unable so soon after a seizure. With just his face bathed in light, he passively watches the screen, well-tucked into the enveloping darkness. He seizes again. A minute later, he stops moving. There is always a slight, peaceful pause at this point. Lost Noise starts, then stops. "YouTube?" I ask again when I think he might be ready.

"I REJECT THAT," I blurt out at Dr. Pink after a particularly scary swoop.

For Pink, medication noncompliance is a moral issue. I get the philosophical position, being a physician myself—the world would be a simpler place if patients just took their drugs. But sometimes I don't want to be sick anymore. I don't want to have what I have or be what I am. The easiest thing to do is not to take medication and to not participate in the daily reminder posed by the supposed remedy.

"Do you know what the natural history of bipolar disorder is?" she asks neutrally.

That neutral disposition is necessary because if I'm challenged with anger, I show my birthright. I was born from a monster. "Maybe?" I respond, wary of where she's going. "We die. Way more often than people with depression. Mortality is very high."

"That's true, but it isn't what I meant. I mean that the natural history of bipolar disorder, how it behaves when it is not treated with medication, is to relapse. Every year, the relapse likelihood increases until, at about five years out, the chance that you'll have relapsed is about 100%."

I choose not to say anything, pretending that I'm invisible.

"It is quite likely that you will die if you don't take medication. Your children will be left without a father."

I choose to perfect invisibility.

"What would not taking medication teach them? You've mentioned to me that you're worried you'll pass on bipolar disorder to them. If they turn out to have bipolar disorder, wouldn't they be less likely to take their medication based on your example?"

A mental image of a generic old Western passes my mind, in which an outlaw on the plains is finally shot by the sheriff. "You got me, pardner," the grizzled hard man says to the straight-backed lawman. "You got me." Then he cinematically expires, expelling a big puff of air until his head falls to the side.

I become visible again. "I see your point."

I LOOK OUT AT THE BLACK TREES limning Exhibition Park, the stars overhead. Janet circles the front of the car and I circle the back, satellites in staggered orbit around our child. I want to walk into the forest and come out starving, pure, with a cure. But the cure is not in the forest, it's back in the car, or where the car will go, or how I'm in the car with the children and with my wife. And how is that? It's hard to keep track of the real world in the flat plains of a separate sadness, the only relief in sight a silo I want to jump from.

CANADIAN HOSPITALS ADOPT A UTILITARIAN STYLE, even children's hospitals. Buffalo Women and Children's is remarkable for its clean, unchipped walls, its high-quality art adorning the corridors. Select areas of the hospital—the foyer, some big donor wings—have the atmosphere of an upscale hotel.

The pre-op area thrills Kaz with its toy selection: cars, blocks, dolls, train tracks. A wall-mounted widescreen television shows an episode of the god-drenched talk show *The 700 Club*. Across from us, a white man and his very white-haired young wife sit in plastic chairs, holding hands while they watch the broadcast. One of the dozen kids on the floor who exponentially expand the toy mess must be theirs. Maybe, like I am, the man and woman are looking for a sign.

Painted on the walls is a continuous mural of an inner city. Smiling children of a rainbow nation (Caucasian, Black, Hispanic, Indigenous, and Asian) play soccer on the street. Smaller kids sit on the shoulders of their dads while others frolic in the shimmering spray from a fire hydrant.

On *The 700 Club*, an elderly yet wrinkleless blond woman reads aloud a viewer's email to a corpulent Pat Robertson. This segment of the show is called Bring It On: Casting Out Demons. "This is an email from Joe," she says. "Joe writes, 'I have liver cancer and was told by my doctor that I have six months to live. But isn't that God's decision?'"

A nurse bends down to Kaz's level and says, "Hey there, young man. I hear you are getting an MRI today. It's very fun. The machine is big. It weighs over ten thousand yous!" Her nametag spells out K-I-R-A in letters made of jellybeans. The other nurses wear blue and turquoise scrubs with designs of boats, stethoscopes, and smiling children, but Kira wears hot pink scrubs with no pattern.

Kaz finds a police car. "Under rest" he shouts at a block. "You in jail!"

On the TV, Pat Robertson fields Joe's question as uttered by the disturbingly tight-faced woman: "Yes it is and all that is, is an estimate and the doctors say, from what we know about medicine that we know the condition of your liver, if things continue as they are, that's what we speculate. On the other hand, they do do liver transplants, I would certainly be looking for one if I were you, you can also be looking for healing, but yes it's god's decision when they take you but I wouldn't discount the prognosis of a doctor but god can tell you something totally different, you will not die and you will live and glorify the lord I CAST THEE OUT, DEMON!"

Why are they not showing cartoons? Kira takes us to a slim man in his early fifties in a small room with a weirdly blue couch. "Hello there Kazoo and Kazoo family!"

Kaz tries to set a Monkeys on the Bed record. How high can he go before he bumps his head? Mama called the doctor...

"I'm the anesthesiologist who will take care of your son today. My name is Dr. A. Everything is happening on time today in the radiology department. I will put Kazoo to sleep, but it will be only deep sleeping." *Bounce bounce bounce.* "He shouldn't need help with breathing unless there's a problem. But if there is a problem, we are ready." Dr. A stops and looks at me directly. "You're a doctor, right?"

Kaz is trying to die now with insane boings. He pretends to have hurt himself: *ow ow ow.*

Cerulean probably mentioned that fact when he filled out the requisition. "Yes," I say. "I'm a doctor."

"Call me James," he says, rubbing his chin.

Pause. Am I supposed to say James right now?

"Let me see if I have this straight. You're from Canada. Your son is two-and-a-half years old. He has new onset focal epilepsy. He has had many seizures that are getting worse with time. And you're here in Buffalo to get an MRI."

"Yes. James."

"Couldn't you get an MRI where you're from?"

I tell James the short version of Cerulean.

It turns out James is Canadian, trained at Queen's. He has practised in Buffalo for over twenty years, leaving the Canadian system because of its delays. "I've seen a lot of people from Canada during my years here. But, man, I didn't know it was this bad." *Bounce bounce ow bounce ow bounce ow.* "Hey, Kazoo, you're going to fall. Doctor says NO MORE MONKEYS JUMPING ON THE BED."

A real doctor in a real white coat to play the game with! Rather than feeling chastened, Kaz is thrilled. *Bouncebouncebouncebounce bouncebouncebouncebounce.* I grab Kaz and sit him on my lap. "No Kaz. That's enough. The doctor's here."

There must have been something menacing in my voice. "Will polices come?" he asks.

"Yes," I respond. "Lots of polices."

Kaz sits very still and smiles at James, who opens a door to the radiology suite. Just outside, a gurney waits. James drops the siderails and says, "Okay, Monkey—get on this bed! We have to go get a special test. Say goodbye to Mom and Dad."

"Dere toys dere?"

"Oh, yes. I play with toys all day. Don't I look like I play with toys? All I do all day is play with kids and toys. You'll see." James and Kaz turn a corner and are gone.

THIS FORM OF WAITING is akin to waiting for seizures to stop: all I want is for my son to come back. A half hour, an hour, then 80 minutes pass. The MRI takes just a few minutes to perform but Kaz needs to be put under, and then he needs to wake up. It takes time to come around from the drugs just like it takes time to rouse after a seizure.

Across from us, the same couple sits, still clasping hands. Like Janet and me, they don't speak. We are like the dead who wait for the dead, like the old people I remember from Catholic church who sat stolidly in pews, serially witnessing transubstantiation, seemingly indestructible until the congregation learned during the Responsorial Psalm that Mrs. Godfearing was in hospital, sick. *Please pray for her. The word of the Lord. Thanks be to God.*

Who knows how long I was back in the past. The couple are no longer here. Where did they go? Which child was theirs? Were their prayers answered?

EVERY MEDICAL SCHOOL features its share of legendary characters, good and bad, no matter the era. Take, for example, the obese respirologist who wheezed while moving from the hospital elevator to the ICU and back. When patients crashed and needed intubation, he always seemed winded, arriving long after students or residents. He would sit down in a chair he pulled over, watching the vital signs readout on the telemetry monitor, trying to catch his own breath.

As a student struggled to get the tube in, he would count down the oxygen saturation level. "91%."

"90%."

"89%."

"88%."

Watching a resident struggle to re-intubate a patient one time, I wondered just how low the number had to go before the respirologist would get out of the chair and help. As hospital legend had it, he had not intubated a patient in years. He never found his breath, and he never helped a critically ill patient find theirs.

"79%."

In the middle of a disaster, don't describe. Just do. Only the fearful have the luxury of description. If BCJ were here, he'd leap to the head of the bed, wield the curved Macintosh blade, progress to the vallecula, and lift forward, elevating Mr. Flappy, the epiglottis, exposing the laryngeal inlet. Transparent lubricant would make the tube slide in like butter.

But BCJ is not a legendary character in hospitals. Only the doctors are granted such status. What is the percentage of my despair?

87%

88%

89%

I call it out, knowing that when it hits 100%, BCJ, being perpetually on call, brutal schedule, will have to make a house call.

ALL I WANT

One of the tricks played upon the mentally ill is to suggest that, since their illness is not objectively quantifiable or even verifiable, they are not sick at all. A reverse logic applies to suicide: why extrapolate to the most extreme outcome in the case of my daughter? Do I envision the worst because I want to cast myself as hero in this story, and not as average father? Or do I see this love story as, instead, a tragic one?

IF ON A WINTER'S NIGHT a traveller were to walk down the Waasis Road in Oromocto, New Brunswick, heading east towards the access point of the Trans-Canada Highway, he would descend into a small depression. Along the north side of the road are tall elms shielding the bungalows from noise. On the south side, a thickly forested hill rises sharply, No Trespassing signs screwed into its trees. As per the paradox, the signs invite trespass but because the signs are marked by the Department of National Defense, no one trespasses (a counter-paradox), including our traveller on this winter's night. Ground marked off in this way might contain the abandoned misfires of previous training games, dud warheads or idiot grenades. Our traveller begins the steeper part of the descent, walking along a simple sidewalk on the south side of the road.

OVER THE PAST TWELVE HOURS, I have been working through what Shneidman calls the dyadic position:

Most suicidal events are dyadic events, that is, two-person events. Actually this dyadic aspect of suicide has two phases: the first during the prevention of suicide when one must deal with the "significant other," and the second in the aftermath in the case of a committed suicide in which one must deal with the survivor-victim. Although it is obvious that the suicidal drama takes place within an individual's head, it is also true that most suicidal tensions are between two people keenly known to each other: spouse and spouse, parent and child, lover and lover. In addition, death itself is an extremely dyadic event.

In this particular case, I identify two dyads, each of which has a directionality. In the parent-child dyad, there is simple grief, apology, and fear. *I am sorry, Zee, that I did not see.* In the child-parent orientation, Zee says to me, *You're not paying attention to me. You don't want me around anymore. You don't. Not really.* In the spouse-spouse dyad, I say to Janet, *This is your fault because you are never around.* Janet says to me, *This is your fault because you gave this to her.*

THE TRAVELLER NOTES THE ABSENCE OF TRAFFIC at two o'clock in the morning in this sleepy model town. He identifies the character of the snowfall collecting on his thick woolen jacket as huge wet flakes, the clingiest kind, stuff children will sculpt into snowmen come morning. The volume threatens to cover everything with a flat white layer. Some distance ahead, who could know how far for sure, an Irving convenience store comes into view, its lights switched off. Indeed, the only illumination for our traveller is provided by streetlights placed at exact intervals. Our traveller counts the steps between poles: ninety-three. He glances up the pole—how many steps to walk to the top? Surely the height of the pole is related to the separation between poles, for the civil engineers of Oromocto were goldilocks, placing long lights a perfect distance apart so that the traveller is never completely in the dark, he merely emerges into a center of clear illumination, travels to a radius of decreasing illumination, and then enters into another circle of increasing illumination until, in turn, he reaches its centre. The street marvellously bright.

ZEE AND I STAND IN THE RECEIVING AREA of Trellis's strip mall office off Silvercreek. Next door, Goody's Restaurant claims to offer the best breakfast in town, that promise baked into their sign. Several empty desks are protected by a thick sheet of glass extending from the reception desk to the ceiling. The glass has a small central hole to allow voice communication. The glass has a sinister cast. Because there is no one to notice, the reception area deserted, I take an inventory of what lies behind. Two photocopiers; five desks derelict with papers; rows of textbooks; flimsy walls that look as if they're made of flypaper.

If a family waits in the forest, does anybody notice? I knock on the glass. No response. "Hello, anybody in there?" I shout through the voice hole. This greeting strikes me as funny, Trellis being a mental health facility.

Stealth attack: the administrative area remains a ghost town, but somehow the facility still knew we were in the reception area. A door at the other end of the hall opens, making Zee jump.

A middle-aged, heavyset woman with shoulder-length brown hair and a puffy face asks, "Stuyonka Neilson?"

Zee looks at me. "Yes," I say. "Call her Zee."

"Hi there Zee. Please follow me. Dad, you're welcome to come in later but I'm going to need to see Zee alone first."

Does Zee want to die? Does she want to get better? Will she even talk today? The woman seems fake nice, offering empathy as a syrup, all sticky and gooey, tasting sweet until one realizes it isn't real and even the scent of it makes one sick. The Nice Lady gently motions to Zee with her hand. My daughter follows her, looking back briefly before turning a corner.

"I'm Shane," I say to Nice Lady's back as she takes my daughter away.

This is a love story this is a love story this is a love story.

They're gone. I sit down, put in earphones, and set the iPod Touch on shuffle.

On the wall are visual reassurances to clientele that they will be okay: posters about domestic abuse, child abuse, substance abuse, bullying, and suicide. Clumsy graphics and awkward text attempt to make it safe for children to speak of what might kill them. Multi-ethnic spherical heads smile on one poster underneath the heading, "We are all able and equal."

No. We are all broken and doomed. I feel trapped, tied to the chair in the bonds of care. This is the second worst moment of my life.

Out in the parking lot, a woman drags a seven-year-old boy from an Escalade. She hauls him by the arm and it takes her whole strength to pull him into the Trellis waiting room. With a strange lack of anger, she shoves him into a chair and sits down herself. I get the impression this is just the degree of force required to make him come. After relaxing her grip, the boy bolts back out the door and the woman chases after him. They don't return. Maybe she feels worse than me. Maybe he does.

Some songs possess the power to disinhibit their listener, uncoupling them from emotional sobriety. The listener cannot help but invest their own longing and hopes into the song's sound. Such listeners hear the song as if it were a hymn, and with such attention that the sense inverts and the song hears them instead, they becomes its instrument.

LCD Soundsystem's "All I Want" begins with a disorganized cacophony progressing to a drum-machine beat that backs a basic organ fingering and a repetitive guitar riff. After a chaotic start, a rigidly repetitive order is eventually imposed. The organ play is crudely competent. The guitar work's rough too. Both components are melodic, but workmanlike, as if a child, learning the basics of both instruments, took what they knew how to do and made a song by looping one idea over and over. James Murphy's voice cuts in next. In a controlled warble, he sings of a girl, a lonely park, and a man.

My mind bends into some nook that, somehow, weaves my daughter's beautiful life into prophecy. When Zee was between the ages of three and eight, our days were spent entirely in parks. We had the choice of Big Park and Little Park. Big Park was further down the road but had more swing sets and play structures. Little Park was closer, less dangerous, and had a higher likelihood of having a friend for her to play with.

But isn't Zee *Zee*, not a mere character in some delusory matrix? There is no prophecy, I am merely mad, lost in this song because I am lost myself. In the chair at Trellis, alone, I pity *myself*. Hearing the first line in the song, I imagine it's *me* walking home from that park without my daughter; in the second line *I'm* looking for a dead girl. Remember the child-parent dyad: *you're* not paying attention to *me*.

To this point, the song's stripped instrumentation and repetitive units provide a scaffold for something extraordinary: a new organ introduces the spirit of my daughter via a vaulting, graceful musicianship that suggests butterflies in a summer field. The melody of the new organ ranges so far, it makes me think of Zee skipping from the park into a forest, where she escapes a witch in a gingerbread house, a wolf in grandma's clothing, and then a troll under a bridge. She dances past terrible things as the organ gets more beautiful, as the melody becomes increasingly intricate and dynamic.

The less difficult beauty does not last. The organ becomes strident, shooting into a higher range, moving the song from a spirit walk in a summer park to something stranger, an aural metaphor for a scream. The song maintains the original base melody but in a slurred, bizarre treatment, as if the organ's keys are being removed with a chisel and pliers. As if psychosis could still be melodic, a more complex beauty, organized nodes of brokenness making the delusion meaningful, even remarkable for its intricacy and structure.

Is Zee talking to the Nice Lady about Big Park, about how she never goes there anymore? Is Zee confessing a plan? We remain in this life, all of us, because of friends, school, activities, and home. What of those do I know of hers? I only know music in a blasted key, and it tells me that I don't know enough.

WHEN THE TRAVELLER REACHES THE LULL OF THE DEPRESSION, he might eventually wonder: what is beyond the penumbra of light encasing the street? Held so safe in the corridor, he might become curious about what could be found on either side of the road. The streetlights stem from the north side, meaning that the south side falls more quickly into darkness. Looking at the forested hill is easy: it stands as one gigantic, rising darkness, with trees blocking out stars until the sky and its cloud fail to be completely dark, illuminated as they are by reflection from the moon. It is the honesty of this darkness that bores the traveller somewhat. He can easily perceive it for what it is: a marked-off wilderness that offers no challenge, excepting the possibility of unexploded military rounds.

MARIANNE, ZEE'S SUNDAY SCHOOL TEACHER, assigns her pupils the usual roles in the nativity play: Jesus, Mary, shepherds, innkeeper, wise men, and Joseph. Oddly, the stiffest competition is for the animal parts: horse, sheep, ass, pig. Zee passively waits until the end, when all the roles are taken by the other children. By default, Zee is named the angel Gabriel.

Each child is responsible for their own costume, meaning of course that their parents are responsible. I hunt the house for a white tunic and sweatpants for Zee, who, surprisingly, already has a stockpile of cardboard, Bristol board, wire, and fancy paper spread out before her.

"Daddies are for getting stuff, and Zees are for making stuff," says the sad girl sitting at the kitchen table. Using the large scissors in her hand, she meticulously cuts the cardboard into wings, then wrestles the wire and gold paper into a halo. More wire goes into a shoulder mount that bears the halo above her head.

Janet's at work, growing cells for her research project, infecting them with virus, making inclusion bodies. If Janet were here, she would help make the angel become even more angelic.

"How big should my halo be, Daddy?"

"Do you want me to google the Vatican's official policy on halo size for angels and archangels?"

Zee makes a face. Not funny.

"Maybe as big as your head," I say.

Do cherubim bear halos disproportionately large, making their little heads droop? Zee carefully wraps the gold paper around the wire until no silver shows through. Sneak attack: "How are you feeling, Zee?"

She keeps her eyes on the halo. "Good."

Sneak attack *fails*.

Zee's name derives from the medieval Slavic word *zdeti*, a word that means "to build, to create." Her halo is delicate and small. "Is there any way I can help you?" I ask.

"No, Daddy. You can't do this, you know. It takes *skill*."

We have a follow-up appointment at Trellis again in a week. Is that soon enough? When will she see psychiatry? Zee sleeps poorly and lately materializes in the master bedroom at odd hours. Sometimes I turn over to see her standing at the edge of the room, silently watching me, a ghostly angel.

IF THE TRAVELLER TRIED TO SEE PAST the streetlights and guardian elms on the north side of the street, however, he faces a challenge. There are, in effect, three walls: two are static and one is in flux. One wall is constituted by light itself, that thrown down by the streetlights overhead. The source is the north side of the street, protecting what is beyond that light source from observation by our traveller, walking as he does on the south side. Another wall is formed by the trees themselves, taller even than the streetlights. Though they have by now long lost their leaves, the thickness of their trunks and their height suggest that the trees are far older than the town, even though the fact seems impossible, as perfectly landscaped as they are on the north side, lining the road in a tightly organized formation. The second wall is constituted by snow, and is dynamic in two ways: descending snowflakes physically block perception beyond themselves, and when they fall heavily, the reduction in visibility is proportionally increased; there is a glare effect from the snowflakes, as mediated by the streetlights, and when the snowflake is perfectly perpendicular with the light, the snowflake casts its greatest glare. Each snowflake falling from the sky is unique and each snowflake in its position in space casts a further unique luminescence based on its specific shape and position in space; the third wall involves simple accumulation of the snow on the bare branches and trunks of the elms.

WHEN ZEE WORKS ON A TASK, she focuses to the exclusion of all else, needing to be pulled from what she is doing else she'll work through supper or long into the night. Small and beautiful things consume her attention—just like her father. "Zee, the halo's done. It's really pretty. Just stop with it, okay? It's perfect."

"But it's not good enough yet."

"Zee, I can't make haloes. Not like that anyway. Your halo is awesome, and it will be the *best* angel halo in the nativity play."

"Daddy, I'm the only angel in the play. So that's dumb."

THE TRAVELLER, HAVING GROWN INCREASINGLY CURIOUS about what exists beyond the veil of light on the north side of the street, pauses, and though no motorists have passed by in the hours of his walk, looks to cross the street, and then crosses, approaching a mounting glare. He might be overwhelmed by the light and get pushed back to the sidewalk where the light is intended to keep him comfortable. But, curiosity proving irresistible on this winter's night, a completely common and unremarkable night unless one is struck by the basic mystery inherent in all things, the traveller persists to the other side, pushing through the threshold of maximal brightness at the base of a streetlight. Further, he steps beyond the elms, which now offer him greater protection from the streetlights. Having been granted another gradated darkness to enjoy, one which deepens with distance, what should he find about fifty feet from the trees but a humped house with a small light on inside, the only light on in what he now recognizes as a street of houses, parallel with the road he was once walking alongside.

ON CHRISTMAS EVE, Zee and I drive to her dress rehearsal at the church. The script's conventional, sticking to the standard nativity story: birth of a child in Bethlehem dutifully foretold by an angel appearing to shepherds, etc. Zee takes her position on steps ascending to the altar. Joseph and Mary sit on either side of Jesus. Bizarrely, Joseph wears a top hat. Mary is swaddled in turquoise blankets wrapped to resemble a nun's habit. Jesus dresses in SpongeBob pajamas and shakes a rattle with both hands. The animals low and graze in front of the stairs with identifying signs draped around their necks: PIG. HORSE. SHEEP. Once the animals finish making their din, Zee lifts her head and intones: "Do not be afraid. We bring you good news of great joy for all people."

First Baptist is lit such that the few parents in the audience sit in darkness. Only the children are visible at the front. Beyond the children, darkness covers where the choir, if this were an actual service, would sing on the right. I sit in the pew furthest back, watching a radiantly somber Zee. When she's done speaking the line, her head declines. When Zee speaks another line, her head lifts and she moves the story forward. Her halo glints, reflecting greater light upon her face. The only thing I know for sure is that what she's saying is not what she's thinking.

When the play is over, everyone forms into a slowly turning circle and bursts into song, the animals having miraculously gained the ability to stand on their hind legs and talk in human voices. Joseph's arm drapes around the nun-ish Mary. The three wise men, all of them girls, laugh as they pull off itchy cotton beards. Zee remains on the steps by herself, her expression blank but her face bright, as if angels shining on high are instructed to keep their distance from mortals.

IF THE TRAVELLER DECIDED TO HEAD TO THE LIGHT, even though he had quite enough light just a minute ago, he would cross a lawn which now wears a thin blanket of snow. Arriving closer still, he would recognize the house as a bungalow, nondescript on a street of bungalows. Closer yet, he would see that the light was shining out of the house's garage. *Perhaps,* the traveller would think, *I am a fool. I am trespassing on this property merely to find a room in which a light was left on, forgotten.* Yet the traveller continues anyway, so close that he must press his face to the small window in the uppermost portion of a door. The traveller is lucky: the window has not yet frosted over. Peering inside, he realizes he was very wrong, the room is remarkable for what it contains. Sitting on an overturned oil barrel is a boy. Near him, several ranks of hardwood are piled to the ceiling. In the far left corner of the room is a woodstove, its heat visible to the traveller shivering outside. The boy, for example, seems comfortable even though he is not wearing a coat. The wood closest to the window bears ice and snow. On a wall are several dozen tools, but organized in no schema the traveller can recognize. The tools seem randomly placed, as if they have been kept from the floor, from chaos and loss, but no more. To find a tool on the wall would not be guaranteed. On a workbench is a sledgehammer and vice grips. The boy has his back to the traveller, so the traveller has the luxury of time, he can really study the scene. The boy, perhaps eight years old, turns slightly, revealing what is on his lap—a pump-action shotgun. The child's mouth is wrapped around the barrel but his arms struggle to reach the trigger. On closer inspection, the action is improperly loaded. The child has not yet managed to get the shell completely inside. But then the child turns back, and from the traveller's vantage point, he sees only a child sitting on a barrel.

Perhaps on this winter's night, the traveller, shocked by the event unfolding before him, tries to intervene. He pulls on the door handle but cannot turn it; he bangs on the door, but realizes that he makes no noise; he punches the glass but his hand bounces off. And yet he knows he cannot witness what is about to happen, that to witness it might make it actually happen, that once the dyad is resolved, the act can be completed. Perhaps the traveller came too far back to what is unalterable and unreachable, something that cannot be healed. Horrified, the traveller turns around on this quiet winter night and retraces his steps.

ONE DAY AS A RESIDENT, I attended an emergency medicine resuscitation seminar. I was ready, having re-memorized Advanced Cardiac Life Support and Advanced Trauma Life Support protocols the week before. My motivating fear spurring attendance was that, when faced with an expiring patient, I wouldn't know what to do.

Looking back, I realize that I didn't know that such scenarios are trick questions of a sort. When something terrible happens to a body, little can be done to stop it and even less can be done to fix it. But the drama for medical professionals is mostly internal, one of knowledge, and in medical education one of demonstrating that knowledge. So I studied in order to be uselessly prepared.

Looking back on the seminar twenty-five years later, the irony is that I remember absolutely nothing about the particular cases, the drugs ordered, the intubations done. I cannot recall a single other person at the seminar, even though I worked with every attendant closely. When not leading a code, all attendants served as resuscitation team members. What I remember instead is that the first ten minutes of the seminar were a complete cold open. After gathering in a room somewhere in the New Halifax Infirmary and waiting for a few minutes after the scheduled start time, the lights went down unexpectedly and a video was shown on a facing wall.

We watched a pilot and a co-pilot chat and drink coffee for the first two and a half minutes. A female voice could be heard speaking off-screen; a flight attendant. The camera's field of view included the back of the pilot's seats and the center portion of their instrument panel, the lateral parts of which were blocked by the seats themselves. A fraction of sky could be observed out the cockpit window, but not nearly enough to provide a full view.

At about the three-minute mark, the co-pilot pointed out an alarm light flashing on the panel. It was a yellow light, and though I am not a pilot, it seemed reassuring that the light was merely yellow and not red. The pilot acknowledged the problem and both pilot and co-pilot began to troubleshoot the causes for the yellow light's appearance. They debated what the signal might mean on a flight that was operating so smoothly, without other indicators of trouble. They tried switching something off, and turning it on again, but the yellow light continued to flash. They tried doing the same thing again, to no avail. To me as an observer, they seemed to really focus on the nuances of what this light might mean much as an internist might debate the relative merits of two comparable drugs. The difference might be a wash, but considering the possibilities is a fun intellectual exercise. By this time, nine minutes and thirty seconds have elapsed in the video, at which point it goes blank.

The lights come up and the physician leading the seminar stands at the front of the room. Somehow he was always there. "So what did you think of the yellow light?" he asks.

Following the rules of medical education, which demand that one answer questions with only correct answers, and because this is a solicitation of opinion which we aren't qualified to give, not being pilots, no one says anything. He says, "The reason the video cut out is because this plane crashed. The video was retrieved in the black box. The point is, you always have information before you. You may even have correct information before you. But never, ever, lose sight of what you're doing along the way. For what is it that you're doing—gathering information? Or are you treating a patient and not a result? If one of the pilots had looked up, had noticed that they were slightly angled to the ground, then everyone on the plane would still be alive because the pilots would have noticed that every other indicator in the plane was failing, and that only the yellow light itself was working, sending a signal that it was somehow in distress."

Shaken by this drama, we stumbled into the rest of the seminar, drugging and shocking patients based on EKG readings, terrified that we were chasing yellow lights in a domain of perpetual alarms.

THE TRAVELLER CROSSES THE THRESHOLD OF LIGHT and is back on the sidewalk. He realizes he must decide in the midst of his otherwise small and unremarkable life, *when should I go.* He has an infinite number of timepoints to go back to (or is it forward?), perhaps too many to choose from, so many that he might postpone the decision, might even, in the torpor of endless choice, live out his life without exercising his power and curiosity. He could, if he wanted to, stop walking entirely. From time to time in the course of the rest of his life, an event might remind him of his power, either through nostalgia or trauma, the former a pleasant recollection of positive experiences and associations, the latter a sudden intrusion into the present of the past itself, the past itself a time traveller.

THE DRAMA OF DEPRESSION IS ENTIRELY INTERNAL. Internal dramas are notoriously difficult to bring to the stage because one cannot dramatize thought or inner conflict. Torpor is not exciting to an audience, and the depressed do not tend towards lively dialogue. Tone presents another problem. Pessimism militates towards Beckettian non-drama: lives held in suspension, the plot one of simply existing.

Should improvement occur, that improvement is gradual, stuttering, a reverse metaphor involving the proverbial frog boiling in a pot. Rather than the water temperature gradually rising until the frog is boiled, in this case the frog is slowly warmed from its frozen state in the hopes that it was merely hypothermic and not dead, that the frog will, once heated to room temperature, hop out of the pot and go on being a frog.

Imagine the cure to a certain kind of depression being love. No drugs are offered, though they are somewhat confusedly sought; doctors are consulted, though they are of little help; appointments are kept out of hope, but their purpose always remains obscure. All that remains is the simple relation between father and daughter, the possibility of igniting that relation into one of healing warmth. As a drama, the story is not dynamic. There is incrementality, dailiness, simple listening and being. There is a dyad of interiority in which the father begins to worry terribly about his daughter, focusing on small details as proof of improvement or of relapse. The tyranny the disorder itself: what is it, and how is it now? Where are we as we move through it? Are we moving through it? When will it be over? Can it be over? Every small experiential detail run through an anxious algorithm meant to descry the moment when—could it be possible—we emerge from the nebula; no, we approach the boundaries of a nebula; no, we realize the nebula has a boundary and that we move towards it; no, we recognize, first, that we are even moving.

Yet there are templates for depressed characters within larger dramas, cultural icons offered to audiences to understand what it is like to want to die without the play itself becoming a Beckettian stasis. I think of these dramas, operating as they do psychologically, as akin to pharmacological treatments of old. Digitalis therapy for patients in heart failure, for example, or warfarin for people with artificial valves. Just a little bit of the poison provides a benefit, but too much and the toxin is lethal. So it is with suicidal characters in imaginative works. They offer the depressed a space to possibly cure themselves. But, mostly, to see themselves, just to be.

WHY THIS ROOM IS FILLED WITH THE SOUND of a thousand sirens, only BCJ can say. *ROOOO ROOOOOO ROOOOOO* resonates, the different pitches of various models asynchronously running to create a sonic wall of the emergency present. I'm bound. I feel leather straps pull my wrists and ankles so that there is no give, not even a slight degree of freedom.

This room is red, but red of a periodic kind, red cast in a circular motion, as if from an emergency light. Like clockwork, I can see the rest of my body, and then I have to wait to see the rest of my body again. Tracking the light on its revolution, but only with my eyes, because I cannot turn my head—these are five points, I realize now—I see Kaz on my right. He is unconscious, drooling, Velcro straps holding him loosely to a board. Further round, I see my father to the left, intubated, bound save for his right arm which points to the ceiling, making rapid little circles, agitating the air.

What did we do to deserve this? The men in this family, all in bondage. One bad, one mad, the other a sadness, a suffering unto Jesus. Above us, BCJ throws a loaded syringe into a dartboard, hitting bullseye. I know the bit from Galatians! *Stand fast therefore in the liberty wherewith Christ hath made us free, and be not entangled again with the yoke of bondage.* But Lord—do you mean all three of us have rejected your liberty? If I could be free, I would take my father from this place. I would carry my son on my back. More than anything else in this life—security; love; comfort—I have wished this: to be free.

Ah. That's better. BCJ slackens my right arm just enough. Soon I will be out of here.

THE EVIDENCE CONCERNING DIVORCE RATES for couples whose child experiences a serious or fatal illness is a glass-half-full situation. If one looks out of windows expecting harm, then the likelihood of harm is what matters. If one looks out to see the sun, then the possibilities that the day brings are what's important. Retrospective studies involving huge pools of data show that the likelihood of divorce is substantially increased. Yet the further time moves out from the illness or death, a survival benefit accumulates—the likelihood of divorce dips below the norm.

Like Kaz does in the pool, I cling to Janet. But I carry her too, by carrying the children. I take the kids to appointments, administer Kaz's medicine, and hold Kaz when the needles come for blood. Part of my waking up is not to escape dreams but also to be shown that, next to me, is the dream come true: the *same* woman, every day, the same children, my children, nearby. The dream is treatment for the nightmare that is the past. I wake to protect these people, to do the best I can as an average father, to not have to one day apologize to Zee and Kaz about an apocalypse in their life, the Armageddon that is a parent not caring for them. I wake to cultivate only the usual regrets, the kind that stick to average fathers. I wake to the same sound, the Canadian flag at Victory Public school whipping in the wind.

Hand makes the belly first, and then I whisper "I love you" to a sleeping body. Janet stretches her arms above her head, arches her back, kicks her legs out straight. "What? Do you want to make love?"

ZEE HEADS INTO THE MINUS-TWENTY SNOW-BLAST for school. A week's gone by since she gave good news of great joy for all people. Now that the Christmas break's over, Zee memorizes dialogue from *Hamlet*. She's been cast as the existential prince, one who provided the wisest advice about philosophy I have ever known.

When Madamester reads an outline to the students, the kids sort into three kinds. Some, like Zee, wish to be characters in the play. Others want to be stagehands—boys to paint and push big things, girls to work cloth and cardboard. A small number of slackers don't want to do anything. "Can we be audience?" they ask.

Amongst the performing set, most of the girls clamour to be Queen Gertrude simply because she is a queen, and queens are, according to Walt Disney's dreamed philosophy, the apotheosis of womanhood. A strange boy who devours paper with "original artworks" of "Umph," a superhero of his own making, aspires to be King Claudius. The roles of Polonius, Laertes, Ophelia, Osric, Rosencrantz, Guildenstern, Horatio, Fortinbras, Francisco, Reynaldo, Voltimand, Marcellus, Bernardo, Cornelius, and Lucianus are picked up easily. Someone wants to play Yorick even though he's just a skull, perhaps especially because he's just a skull. No boy wants the role of Hamlet because playing him means too much memorization.

At the moment in her life when Zee was actually living the play's lines "You cannot, sir, take from me any thing that I will more willingly part withal—except my life, except my life, except my life," she agrees to play Hamlet. Everyone knows she's smart enough to pull it off, is the obvious choice.

Except my life except my life except my life.

With the performance date for Hamlet fast approaching, Zee reads through the script each evening. She prefers for someone to listen to her lines. She hits the notes now, emoting through the text; she's *good*.

In a week she no longer needs the script to cue. Zee prances around the room, playing her part. Behind me, Burning Crown Jesus benignly watches us from the window, making us feel safe. I know he enjoys Zee's performance. He knows I know. When she reaches the end of Act One, the scene where grown men see and talk to ghosts, I join her and say in a silly Elizabethan accent, "There are more things in heaven and earth, Horatio, than are dreamt of in your philosophy." It's the only time I see her make a faint smile.

I know BCJ is grinning behind us, though. He's really on our side, cheering us on, our number one fan. Rarely, Zee scurries back to her script, afraid she'll flub and freeze during the real performance. "I'll ruin the play, Daddy," she says dejectedly. "It will be all my fault."

Her enunciation of all my fault is HUGE, LANGOROUS. Aaaaalllll. Myyyyyy. Faulllllt.

"You have the big role, Zee. But Madamester made you Hamlet because she knows you can do it. If you make a mistake, that's okay. Besides, isn't Jacob supposed to whisper out lines from behind the curtain if anybody forgets?"

"Yeah," Zee says, unconvinced.

We see Nice Lady every two weeks now, spaced back from every week. As more time passes, I get the sense that the feeling is bleeding off, that the destructive resonance is decreasing. Not gone, but receding. Zee wanted to die for a good two months, I know this. But the desire is fading.

LOSING COUNT OF ADMISSIONS, dose increases, YouTube clicks, and futile prayers, I'm reduced to an awareness of only one unit of time: the duration of seizure. But as the gaps without seizures increase, another unit of time begins to shape my days: seizure-free time.

ABBA-Cadabra is on the stage, two women and two men, a high-grade tribute act performing in a Toronto hotel. Dressed in flowing white uniforms, the women are preposterously gorgeous. The brunette sports a white blouse and a deep v-cut showing a crevasse of cleavage, and the blonde is barefoot. Both women wear wreaths in their hair. The two average men bare hirsute open chests. Bjorn, the taller man, says to Benny, the smaller one, "To sell millions of records, hire beautiful women to sing. Easy. Right Bjorn?"

The small one winks at the audience and says, "You are naughty, Benny." Bjorn turns to Benny and says impishly, "We should hire two more!"

Benny smiles at the audience and replies, "Really, ladies and gentlemen. Agnetha and Anni-Frid are married to much richer men than us. They just let *us* appear on stage with *them*. We're their creatures."

Wreathed Agnetha and Anni-Frid bang tambourines against their thighs, keeping the beat. They are packaged to appear as ditzy goddesses, brainless bimbos. Their arch smiles belie the lie. Anni-Frid leans into the microphone to deliver the punchline, "To sell millions of records, find two guys and tell them what to do. Easy! Right, Agnetha?"

Kaz is big-eyed, too small to articulate complex thoughts, but if I had to guess from his expression, he's thinking something like this: *I fell asleep in a hotel room. How did we go from there to this huge stage?*

"Yes guys. We are ABBA-Cadabra," Benny says to the assembled audience of veterinarians and vet technicians. "Agnetha and Anni-Frid are happily married in North Vancouver. We're as upset about it as you are. They've got two kids each." I look at the crowd and recognize, for perhaps the thousandth time in my life at vet events, that it is overwhelmingly female.

Agnetha says, "Benny and Bjorn are bachelors, ladies, and probablyyyyy lifelong. Tracks, right? But one of you out there could change that, I'm sure. *I* certainly wouldn't recommend it, though."

The ABBA-Cadabra event marks the end of the veterinary conference. Kaz and I did High Park and the Beaches earlier in the day. Yesterday, we spent our time at a giant indoor bouncy castle activity camp. Now he slips from his mother's lap, bleary-eyed and mystified, and walks in front of the copycat band. He is the very first to take to the dance area.

Bjorn laughs. "Hey, how are you doing tonight sir?" Bjorn says to my son, his banter coming over a muted, extended intro to "Dancing Queen." Kaz doesn't respond. He's *concentrating*, watching stagecraft.

"Sir, are you okay? You look like you've had a little too much milk to drink tonight." Kaz's mouth is open, his head tilted upward. "I do think this young man will need some help up here. We are about to play a song and he shouldn't have to dance alone. We will call your mother to you. We know how to do that." Bjorn looks supremely confident.

"Bjorn knows about mommies," Agnetha says, undercutting him, hitting that tambourine against that perfect thigh, her white smile razzing Bjorn with obvious affection.

Wait. These people must be married to one another. They're just too *on*.

Dancing Queen's ambient melody gets a little louder, closer to breaking the surface. "Sir, do you like to dance?" Bjorn asks.

Kaz looks at Janet. Taking this as a nod, Bjorn says, "Marvellous."

Speakers pump out the sound of the two wreathed angels. Benny bops, playing piano notes ostentatiously between their chorale.

Bjorn is right. Few in the audience resist. Janet gets up to dance with Kaz, forming part of a growing crowd on the dance floor. At the end of the song, and now with people pressed in front of them, participating, ABBA-Cadabra double down on the impersonation. Bjorn banters about a show in Bern that went up in flames last week; the sound stage's power system blew out three songs in, and the crowd rioted. "Don't you guys get any ideas," Bjorn says, making everyone groan.

Agnetha complains to Bjorn that she can't take the fame, she wants to retire to Richmond Hill with some ordinary guy. "I mean, how hard can it be to find one?" she says, staring Bjorn down.

Janet holds Kaz's hands, trying to get him to move. She's his Dancing Queen, just as Bjorn predicted. But Kaz is stunned. Against this wall of music, of show, he takes in as much as he can, observing. Janet waves his arms, making him sway, but cannot break the spell. Agnetha and Anna-Frid move to the front of the stage and smile at my unmoving son. It feels like Agnetha and Anna-Frid sing just for him, and perhaps they are, for Kaz is one month seizure-free.

THE TRAVELLER IS NOT THE SORT OF PERSON who is moved by nostalgia, being of a cold cast of mind. He has little to be nostalgic about, and to judge him on his lack of nostalgia would be to deny him his past, and thereby strip him of his power to return to the past. Perhaps the traveller, in the midst of his regular duties on a nondescript day, or a day of great and terrible import, a traumatic day that by its nature *as* trauma contributes to another inexhaustible store, in this case of unresolved difficulty, decided to go back to a moment when everything went wrong, perhaps a path not taken if we are speaking of the mildest possibility, or perhaps a maiming, or loss of a key relationship, be that romantic or filial, or a ruinous financial loss, or an irresistible pattern of poor decisions such as that constituted by addiction; perhaps the traveller wishes to return to a single one of these and attempt to resolve the trauma, or maybe to review whether it was really as significant as his current self thinks.

I WANDER INTO THE SMALL VICTORY GYMNASIUM. Empty chairs sit in orderly rows. A thick red curtain is drawn over the stage. The gym walls are covered in students' pictures of skating rinks, Zambonis, snowmen, and Santa Claus. There is a central explosion of snowflakes on the east wall, each one carefully cut. Other parents file in and take their seats.

I lose track of time from then on. Laertes and Hamlet cross swords. Time disassembles again as I walk Zee home. I hear Santa-bearded Polonius's words in my head. *I have a daughter I love passing well.* This thought gets sticky. *I have a daughter I love passing well I have a daughter I love passing well I have a daughter I love passing well.*

DOES THE TRAVELLER WISH TO BE A WITNESS TO HIMSELF, to watch the infliction of a historical wound, so that he can better understand the manifestations of current pain and their ramifications? Perhaps he knows that he will be somehow frustrated by the lack of consummation of that which he is looking for, his memories playing tricks on him, having changed colour over the years, eliding details, emphasizing others. He decides to jump back to the past as if leaping from a balcony rail, possessed of the intent to warn his past self, or to prevent his past self from making the poor choice that becomes forever determinant of future sadness.

"I DON'T NEED TO SEE YOU FOR A YEAR, since the seizures have stopped," Cerulean says. "Most of the time when medication works, the seizures don't come back and all that's required is blood work and adjusting doses as the child grows."

But something remains wrong. I know this. Something is not explained. Kaz is not like other children. He is uncoordinated. He misses social cues. He seems to melt down more than other boys his age. "I think there is something still wrong," I say. I don't know why, but all this time, with Kaz being struck down and having an obvious disaster with obvious test results explaining that disaster, I still believe we are chasing a yellow light. Inside, I feel that something's not right.

Cerulean looks at his watch. "Wrong?"

"Yes. Kaz seems behind to me."

"Well, the seizures would do that, right?"

"No. He's always seemed behind."

"Can he do up his own zipper?"

"What?"

"On his winter coat. Can he do up his own zipper?"

"It takes him a few minutes. Most of the time I have to do it for him. But yes, he can do it, if given enough time."

"Well, that's a key milestone. If he can do it, then he's developing normally. There's no need to worry."

Janet looks uneasy too. Kaz tries to climb into Cerulean's toy box, but is too large to fit, the lid won't close over top of him. "Maybe we can see you sooner than a year, in case we have additional concerns," she says.

"I'm not sure it's possible," he says. "My schedule is packed. But I will check in with Lemontine to see."

GIRDED AGAINST THE ELEMENTS like a prepared, experienced traveller, he walks up the hill for hours, eventually reaching a bridge that he crosses, somehow resisting the urge to climb over its rail and plummet to the Saint John River below. After successfully crossing the bridge, the traveller walks farther, along the river, without streetlights or sidewalk, on rough roadside, at risk of being mowed down by oncoming motorists. If struck, this would be another way of saying it is too difficult to return to the past, too dangerous, that the physical laws of this world preserve us, they keep us safe, held in the cradle of our traumas that are too catastrophic to revisit.

STUFFED FULL OF RELIGIOUS REMNANTS, I remember words to prayers but have no reason to say the words. They are just names—dead names. I'm trained to say the names. But how can they help me now?

We get better by realizing that other people love and need us. In Christianity, an assumption is the bodily whisking of a human from earth to heaven—a kind of proof that God has always been listening and, when the time is right, he takes us. We always assumed he was. Zee sees doctors, her pastor, her teachers, her family. Light, and gladness, and joy, and honour. We see her, we listen. But I think we didn't see her for a while. We stopped listening.

"Zee, did you want to stop skating for a while, or maybe go less, just once a week maybe?"

"No."

"I was thinking it might be a good idea. Maybe you're too busy?"

"No."

"Well, is there anything you think we could reduce? I think you're too busy."

"I'm not too busy, Daddy. You're too busy. Before you took this vacation, *you* worked forever! Sometimes I skate and no one watches! I'm out there for two hours you know! And I was coming home in the dark! It was *scary*."

There is satisfaction in being good enough, the same kind of satisfaction Jesus takes in his new phase. But there is no satisfaction to be taken in not being good enough, in being derelict.

THE TRAVELLER ALWAYS HAS THE OPTION TO STOP, to say a safe word, one like Hallelujah, in the falling snow. He can sing to the snow and marvel how the matrix of flakes is not dense enough to absorb sound. In this sense he is singing to himself, and in doing so, he may resolve that he is of this world, that these are his acts of self-care. The traveller becomes the apostle Paul, ministering just after the death of Jesus Christ, he who died for our sins, he who sponsored our eternal life. The catastrophe healed, in snow. None of this makes any sense, except in a closely contained world, the snowflakes connecting to one another, little nodes of meaning that glow benignly, that suggest the traveller no longer needs to keep on the journey, he can rest. The traveller, though, at his peril, needs to complete the pilgrimage. He must see this through.

ARE PARENTS AND CHILDREN DOOMED to perpetually try to get ahead of some ancestral monster that pursues us? If yes, can our lives still be called free? Should I free myself from monsters by focusing on the future, on faith? Another father standing in a field might remember playing there with his daughter a few years prior and think: *we should play here again.* Since my children fell ill, I stand in fields and playgrounds, gymnasiums, and church classrooms and have the same thought, but with an accompanying counterthought: *we may never play here again.* Some of the fields aren't there anymore. Maybe the fields have forgotten the children. Maybe the children have forgotten the fields.

Threat imposes a different chronology. Threat teaches that there is only so much time to be loved in this world. Threat casts compromised light upon memory. Threat does not diminish these memories, but it alters the mood of their recollection. If I make too much of too little, of looking at a little girl with a butterfly net in a field or a little girl on a scooter or a little girl singing a song, or if I clench my fists as my son seizes on the ground and feel that he's dying, then such is the enterprise of making sense of a mystery or certainty or lie or prophecy that, once given enough time, I will still not understand. Shone in the proper light, memory is an open, prayerful mouth.

IF THE TRAVELLER WAS LEFT UNMOLESTED by vehicular traffic, if he walked the three days and nights required to arrive at his destination, an ever-eastwarding that in time became a southward walk, moving from one Canadian province to another, from near the capital of one Canadian province to the capital of another; if he had the strength to do this, the energy, and the provisions required; if the traveller did not stop moving, never slowing or ceasing his stride, continuously moving through the flow of time as time itself elapsed—then, perhaps, time would deem him worthy of his chosen experience, the one he ultimately decided upon from a host of such memories, from a bountiful trove. Quite possibly, the physics of the world would relax and grant him an audience with himself, albeit briefly. The arduousness of his journey and his dedication would impress upon the cosmos that on this winter's night, a traveller would, at long last, realize where his entire life has been returning to, that it would disclose this secret.

OUR TIME WITH NICE LADY COMES TO A CLOSE. Zee is better. Yet I have decided to play things out to the end. Who knows? There may yet be a safeguard to be won. After a time of five months—long after it was required, and occurring long distance—it's time to meet the T-man.

T-man's a doc in a box, a boob tube shrink. The child psychiatrist's image is beamed in from a telemedicine conference room in London, Ontario. His thick hair cut short, with a black beard enough to make Freud afeard, he mans a grey desk with odd holes drilled into its surface.

He says, "Hello there. Hello Stonka. How are you today?"

Zee looks down at the ground. "Hello T-Man," she says.

"She's Zee," I say.

"Zee, are you comfortable talking to me, an actual real person, but a real person on the television?"

"Yes," Zee says.

Pleased, he turns his attention to Nice Lady. "Hello again," T-man says. Keeping his gaze on Nice Lady, he adds, "Hello, Sir Dad. Now I will talk to Zee privately. That's the best way to begin."

Since I was provided no opportunity to object, Nice Lady escorts me to my usual seat opposite the WE ARE ALL ABLE AND EQUAL poster.

I disagree again. We aren't *all* able. Maybe none of us are able. I just want us all to *be*. I want the slogan, and the larger world, to be WE ARE ALL. I slip away from time again.

Nice Lady's face reappears in the doorway. She ushers me back into the room. Each step back creates a mini-vacuum of anger. I had to wait five months for this, I'm ready. I already know what T-man will say. He will summarize that Zee is now at little risk, that he hesitates to make a diagnosis at this time, that he will let us go and wish us well, that things look good right now—platitudes that I might myself offer, were I in his situation, things I've even said to parents before. But I would have said such things not knowing what I know in this case, that my family history suggests otherwise, that this difficulty may recur.

T-Man follows the suspected plan to the letter. "Zee is doing well now. What you've done for her is working. Keep it up. You should be proud of her. She's come a long way." I am supposed to rejoice? The doctor says my daughter is better. The system has made me wait until it could offer nothing. *Come a long way*? I think. *To hear you say goodbye to her?*

I look over at Zee. "Did you tell the doctor the truth?" I ask.

T-Man nods most forcefully on Zee's behalf. He wears a gobbly smile. "Oh yes, Zee and I had a very frank discussion."

"My question's for Zee," I say. This is my time for reckoning, I won't have the floor wrested from me. Zee stays quiet. "Zee, did you tell the doctor *how* you planned to die?" Zee wouldn't tell anyone that, not me or Janet or Nice Lady. Our hope was that she didn't have an actual plan at all.

Except my life except my life except my life.

What do I have to lose, anyway? Except Zee, of course. Except everything.

Zee slumps in her chair. T-Man isn't smiling or bobbing his head anymore. "Yes, Stonka?" he asks. Fuck, isn't it his job to find out this shit on his own?

"I'll ... get a knife. I'll cut my neck. Maybe cut off my head ... maybe." Everyone in the room knew this was a child's conception of a method; furthermore, each of us knows that Zee wouldn't do that now. But she might have stumbled into something like that around Christmas. And she might stumble into it again.

"Can I speak to you without Zee in the room, T-Man?" I ask, thinking of the many glittering knives in our cutlery drawer. Steak knives. Bread knives. Paring knives.

Nice Lady takes Zee out and sits with her.

"Stonka is better, she's low risk right now," T-man says.

"I am aware that Zee is better, thank you," I say as coldly as I can, my hands folded in front of me on the boardroom table, mimicking T-man's posture. "My concern is the future."

"Of course she might get sad again," he says. "But you'll just have to bring her back and we will reassess her."

I repeat what I said to Nice Lady on our second visit: a roster of bipolar illness turning our family tree a bright, burnt orange, finishing with the story of Andrew, my cousin, dead at age fourteen, hanging from that family tree, an oration fueled by a passionate desire to tell T-man, in addition, to go fuck himself.

T-Man makes *his* move. "I want to make sure of something," he says. "Are you currently on medication yourself?"

"Of course I am, T-man. I am officially crazy. Practically diagnosed, even."

He requires further verification. "What drugs?" he asks.

"Lithium and Abilify," I say.

Perhaps I am confabulating. He must check. "What doses?" he asks.

My my my. Am I fibbing? Let me see. "Lithium 600 mg b.i.d. and Abilify 10 mg q.h.s," I respond, mimicking his gobbly smile. "Did you want to know what it's like to be in five-point restraints, too? Or maybe you're curious about having a trauma run on you in the same emergency department you worked in the day before, because you jumped off a building."

Silence. Maybe we are in a metaphorical restraint right now, the both of us?

T-man budges a little. "You're a doctor, right?" He talks about medication, itemizing the stepwise rungs of drug therapy for children. I knew this rundown already, and drugs aren't what I want for Zee. Drugs aren't what she needs. Apparently, T-Man and I don't understand one another, a dysfunctional doctor-dad dyad.

"I don't want a diagnosis or a drug," I say. "I want a psychiatrist Zee can see on a regular basis, in London or closer. I want Zee to have a doctor she can talk to, a doctor able to help mentally ill kids. I know that having such a doctor, a doctor who will listen to the truth, is saving."

T-Man is in the television, though. There's a reason for this, as well as a reason for why it took so long to see him. "I'm sorry, I'm just doing this telemedicine consult. I can't see your daughter on an ongoing basis."

"Can anyone else in London see her?" I press.

"There is a doctor here—but—well, there is a doctor but I think they can't see any more cases. There is a clinic, but you'd have to go through their screening process, and your daughter doesn't meet criteria—it doesn't make sense that you'd even come to London to—"

T-man proceeds to tell me a truth that is not saving. It is a truth I know well, but it's only a partial truth. He says, "Dad, the evidence is that we can't prevent suicide. For example, admissions don't make a difference on the number of completions." Diagnosis by this average father: not a People-Who-Care. What if the people professionally responsible for my children could just give one single shit?

And it's over. "Thank you," I say. Zee and I leave together. As I walk out the doors, the light hitting my face, I understand a fuller truth: showing you care as a physician makes all the difference in the world, both in heaven and on earth.

SO NEAR TO HIS DESTINATION, the traveller succumbs to nostalgia, lured by the place he finds himself, a city of his long-ago past that contains many pleasant memories in addition to the one that is his true destination. If the traveller slows to contemplate these memories and their nested relations, perhaps feeling an urge to deviate from the path, to walk to the waterfront or to a small vale on College Street, then the great powers that determine the means of time travel, the ones who guard the gate, would whisk him back to his present, unharmed, but also to the moment of his triggering, and the arduous journey would all be for naught—the assumption thwarted.

WHEN ZEE FELL ILL, what I believed in became odder, stretched, until I was forced to take pleasure in the smallest of things, the rationale being that detail is where meaning accrues. I came to believe in the sound of her footsteps and the lovely detritus on her dinner plate. Every word Zee speaks, the time she goes to bed, whether she wants to play with a friend—all of these become factual strands in a cobweb of meaning, my constitutive paranoia investing detail with unreasonable significance. Grasping at straws, I may break the straws.

Religions acquire depth in paradox. Getting better relies on paradoxical logic too: I need to spend time with Zee, but I also have to cease my relentless exegesis of her life.

At the kitchen table, with my head resting on my hands, I listen to Zee play piano. She moves through the major key songs too briskly, her head held at ninety degrees, the level position that is so elusive to her when she figure skates. Moving to a song in the minor key, her head droops. She slows down and makes fewer mistakes.

I ask, "Why do you like the sad songs more than the happy songs, Zee?"

Maybe this is the kind of question that'll trick her into talking about her feelings.

Zee surprises me. "Maybe it's *you* who like the sad songs more, Daddy."

IF THE TRAVELLER STAYS TRUE TO HIMSELF; if he continues, relentless, across the city, over the Angus L. Macdonald Bridge, and, taking North Street, and from there a series of streets that are automatic to him, unimportant, mere repetitive passages he once took without a thought, impatient to travel to hospitals, or to a girlfriend, or home, the place he had just came from, even though to think of the place he had just come from as home would be troubling to him, jarring, as if this was a realization that was overwhelming, somehow out of place itself; then, soon, our traveller arrives on Summer Street, a place of austere beauty in the winter, again, like the previous place, one featuring trees that slightly lean over the street, bearing branches heavily laden with snow, a sleepy and melancholy place that, in other circumstances, might induce feelings of paralytic nostalgia, a desire to slow his stride and enjoy, for but a moment, its perfection, but which now only serves to quicken his stride. If, on this winter's night, the traveller deems the terrain conducive to running, then he would run, even though he feels exhausted from the long journey. He might be late, or too late.

ONE SUNDAY THE CHILDREN in the younger Sunday school class at First Baptist make paperclip angels again. The paperclip requires a few bends until distinct wings project out from the central section. Lashed to the back of the angel is red string for colour and grip. Contorted at the top, the paperclip gives the appearance of a round head or halo. Zee hands two crafty angels to me, red and pink. "I made them today, Daddy. Guess what they are."

"Are they angels?" I say.

"Yes. You're supposed to hang them from the car mirror," she says.

We walk out to the car from the church. I suspend a red angel from the rear-view mirror and safeguard the other angel in my pocket, a little ceremony involving only me and Zee. On the walk home, Zee tells me, "Teacher says that when you see it, you're supposed to think of God." But whenever I look at it, I think only of Zee.

THE TRAVELLER TURNS THE CORNER on South Street and takes a few more steps down Summer Street, much less wooded, much less beautiful, a long series of tenements extending on both sides into the distance. He turns again and enters a parking lot large enough to contain just a few cars, maybe only enough for the tenement's residents, the traveller is unsure but cannot deviate from his intent, cannot turn his gaze to properly count, he only registers that this is the place he must be, that he is very near now. The traveller ascends the wooden staircase adjacent to the lot, one rising up to a third floor, each step steady even though the traveller, rather than exhibiting his previous hurry, now wishes to slow down, gird himself, prepare, even though he knows that to do so would break faith and terms. The traveller doesn't stop or slow, but instead presses on, his tread stamping down the snow that continues to fall. He walks a path he had taken over two thousand times, so long ago, but which is now one more in number.

ZEE'S ON COMPETITIVE ICE—no more Star A or Star B, she's with the big kids. To be able to skate in this session, an axel is the minimum requirement. Most of the other skaters are in high school. Maggie, the obvious champion, is working on her triple toe loop.

The Sleeman Centre speakers are quiet. The Guelph Storm clock says 6:02 AM. Janet and Kaz sleep in the marital bed. In just the past two months, Zee's skating has exploded in terms of technique: axel, then double salchow, then double toe loop. She runs up and down the rink stairs before skating, preparation her coach demands she do unsupervised—in total, half an hour of stairs and skipping before even lacing up skates.

Out on the ice, a dozen young women whirl and perfect the current challenge while approaching the next: maintain the axel but prepare to do a double; maintain the double but prepare for the double combination; maintain the combination but work towards a double axel. Landed the double axel? Then be like Maggie. Try a triple.

I don't know how to tell the difference between the kind of jumps Zee does. They are all so fast. After practice, she asks, "Did you see my double toe?"

"I can't tell. You seem to be in the air longer, and moving faster."

"Arrgh. Daddy, if I can learn how to do the jumps then you should be able to learn how to tell what they are. I mean, what's harder?"

"Well, I know if you land on your butt that means you were trying to get the double toe, right? Because you start facing front and you hit your landing leg going backwards. I can't tell if you land it though. Just if you don't."

"Daddy. You've got to learn. I really want you to see."

After practice one day Zee complains she landed three double toes and I didn't even smile. I tell her, "Do gang signs when you land the double toe. That way I'll know!"

After ten minutes of on ice warm up, just edge work and stretching, she starts on her jumps. Momentum, jump, fall. She doesn't look up at me. Whenever Kaz watches Zee do jumps, he tries to leap as far as he can, falling forward. Sometimes he throws his arms out and spins around, eventually falling on his backside. "123 Jumpers!" he warns us when it'll be a Super Big Jump, and we move Very Far Back. Backer. Backer.

Momentum, jump, land, but no gang signs. Must have been an axel.

Momentum, jump, land. Her left and right hands, both gloved, go near her face. She waves them doing a double V sign, bending and straightening her knees. She made the double toe!

Jump, gang signs. Jump, gang signs. Jump, gang signs. The Rink Moms look at Zee, then at me. I do gang signs too. Who cares! Momentum, jump, gang signs. The speakers blare Rihanna's contralto, the singer's sharp tone cutting against the ice.

THE TRAVELLER RECOGNIZES that he must heed the speed he has been assigned. To slow down cancels the journey, according to the governance of this process; but to hurry is, in a sense, to skip past the journey, to disregard the process and thereby disrespect it. The traveller cannot force the return to the scene of his memory, for the nature of the memory itself is that it has always taken its time. It occurred in time, and took its own time to do so; it is situated in that stream, and flowing from that moment is the cataclysm, an unfolding series of effects that influenced the traveller's life thenceforth. To hurry to this experience only puts it beyond reach, inaccessible to those of unalike spirit. To gain admittance to a place and time, one must reconstitute oneself. One must be of that place and time.

DR. PINK ASKS, "Are you sleeping?"

"Yes." (No.)

"How is your concentration?"

Good. *(It isn't.)*

"Are you having thoughts of suicide?"

"No." *(I am.)*

"Has your weight changed?"

"No." *(I've lost twenty pounds.)*

"How is the paranoia?"

"The same." *(It's worse, which is why I'm answering questions like I am.)*

"Like how?"

"People are doing things to me on purpose."

"What people?"

She doesn't understand. She never does when I tell her how the world is interconnected, how meaning is made from the tiniest mote.

"Shane, you really should consider a medication to help with the paranoia. If you don't, it could become sticky—hard to get rid of."

But it's been here so long and provides me with such a chorus of insight—why would I want to be rid of it? What if it is the only kind of love I have in the world, the love of things and people and how they are all related?

"No thanks, Pink. I'll keep taking the lithium, though."

IF ON A WINTER'S NIGHT A TRAVELLER raised his gaze, for his habit in this past he now finds himself reliving was to look down, to ensure his footing was secure, to not slip and fall on the steep stair, then he would find no light shining from within the uppermost apartment. Further, his path is unlighted. He is right to look down, to scan for ice and obstacle, but he grants himself one deviation from the protocol, one desperate difference, and prays that the gods who author this process grant him the same mercy he grants himself, that he may be permitted to take just a few more steps, to make the final landing.

RATHER THAN SHIP HER OFF TO CAMPS, I take care of Zee over the summer to solidify her recovery. "Milkweeds!" Zee sings. I stop the car. She's out before me. By the time I get to the plants, she's finished with the leaf tops and is looking at the underside in case any caterpillars are hiding. Rather than look for the insect, I watch her intense focus, her systematic scanning. Her hair's tied back in a ponytail; she wears pants, to prevent pricking and thorning. All business.

Back in the car we go, moving along highway 124.

"Milkweeds!"

I stop again. This patch is bigger, with work for me to do. I scour for caterpillars, but the result is the same—no luck.

"The Caterpillars HATE me!" Zee shouts, happy.

We've driven all day, trying highway 4, then York Road; now to Cambridge we go. Zee knows this will be our last attempt until we go again tomorrow, but it's getting late in the summer. Another possible explanation for our lack of success: our neighbour, an immigrant from Barbados, says the city sprayed and sprayed for twenty years and now Guelph has trouble attracting monarchs even though the city stopped spraying a half-decade ago. "We're reaping the consequences of environmental rape," Zee quotes back to me, chagrined that there's nothing to find today.

Father and daughter seek a monarch caterpillar that could be crawling on a single plant in a ditch or amidst a field of milkweed. When three milkweeds come into view at the side of the road, each clearly suffering from the proximity, Zee immediately becomes energized.

"Milkweeds!"

The nights are slightly colder now, the sun with smaller catchment. Zee's found scores of tuft moths so far on this trek, also thousands of strange red bugs that congregate together in copulative clutches. In the mornings, dozy yellowjackets sip water from the milkweed's decanter, making monarch-hunting somewhat dangerous.

On one of the plants, I spot a single bulbous monarch. Do I pretend not to see it and try to direct Zee this way? I reach for the chartreuse slug-like crawler with black markings, careful not to knock it off the plant. Zee's turning a leaf over on another plant. "Monarch!" I sing. Zee takes the monarch and lets it march up her arm; then she moves it to her other arm. The monarch likes to climb, but not to descend.

"My Monarch Caterpillar," she says. "I name you Monarchy."

When Zee was three years old, she loved things with wings. That night the caterpillar we caught forms a cocoon, probably out of shock; three weeks later, we find nothing but a punctured shell, having left the top off the monarch's glass container. "The monarch is better off free, Daddy," she insists.

IF THE TRAVELLER DOES NOT FALL, nor is whisked back to his present by his recklessness, then he stands in silence on the landing as the snow falls. He looks out at the night, the city sloping down to the water; he is not stopping his journey, indeed he continues on it as per the contract, for this is exactly what he would do if he were back in this past time living it for the first. Back then, he would regard the city and marvel at its several hundred thousand souls, at the collective but individual struggle, and, of course, at how desperately he wanted to end his own. If the traveller turned to his left, he would see the sliding glass doors that he opened perhaps ten thousand times in the past, perhaps twenty; doors that are a quotidian part of existence but, according to the laws of the universe that we are all subject to, including the traveller, doors that can yet become portals into the most disruptive and terrifying moments of life.

THE PARISH OF ST. VINCENT DE PAUL rests on the midpoint of a hill, the adjacent graveyard providing the necessary gravitas. The parking lot is full thanks to the nostalgia of Christmas Eve service. Here at mass in my home church, the place I'd been baptized and confirmed, where I prayed for the dead as a child and where I thought of my own death as relief, I learned the healer and poet's mutual function best: enumerate the sick and dying. Back then I didn't know that poetry and doctoring are, at bottom, responsorial psalm: *Lord let us pray* after the names of the dead and dying are called. The names keep coming, there's no stopping them. But there is time enough to say them respectfully, and time enough to listen.

Roman Catholicism is an orgy of death as paradox: death as life, life as death, death in life and life in death. Dutifully, perhaps too fervently, I prayed for the names I didn't know, the sick and dead names. These prayers moved seamlessly into the priest's recitation of the Eucharist.

Zee and I sit together in a pew three rows from the back, near the Ninth Station of the Cross, the one where Christ falls for the third time. As we walked in, Zee was handed a carol book, twenty songs to be sung during the service, her new recruitment in the Catholic church, a full year after her role as angel in a Guelph protestant church.

Father W is new, the latest of a wave of priests since my confirmation. He's thin, short, and near retirement. He wears the same green vestment that I remember from long ago, throwing the same holy water with the same mace, standing at the same altar. He sings with a homely voice, a low and thin warble that clashes with the choir, a choir that's improved from the one of my memory. His hands have the tight, stiff features of scleroderma.

Father presides over a revised mass. Responses are changed, prayers are different—how long has it been since I've been? Changing these words is like rewriting the commandments to articulate a different faith. I can no longer say "And also with you" but must say, instead, "And in your spirit." To my ears, the Apostolic Creed is now lessened, the meter of poetry drained from of it. What does the priest mutter as his aside to God when he stands over the body and blood of Christ? Then again, I too say different things to Zee now, more important things. Maybe it's right that the Catholic Church renovates its prayers.

My daughter sings the Christmas songs on the program that she knows. An impaled wooden Christ—the same one from my childhood—surveys the faithful. There is no Christmas play in this church, and there had never been in all the years I attended. No Children's Time, nor had there ever been when I was growing up—children were segregated in a separate, glassed-in room. We could see the service but couldn't disturb it. God was protected from us.

Here I stand on Christmas Eve in a Holy Roman Catholic Church, flagship faith of global conservative Christianity. Once upon a time, I looked out the window as a child into the church proper, at gold and stained glass and grainy woodwork. Once upon a time, I dipped my hands in holy water as men, women, and other children also immersed their hands.

Father W speaks The Prayer of the Faithful, that roll call of the dead. Women I never knew are dying, some already gone. "This Christmas, we are to pray for them," Father W instructs.

"Lord, hear our prayer," the congregation drones.

The priest adds an unusual piece once the names are read: "And pray for all those who grieve this night."

"Lord, hear our prayer."

The Catholic Church is now praying for the living and not just the dead and dying? Communion begins. The faithful start into "Hark, the Herald Angels Sing." Suddenly compelled, I stand up and join the communion line, taking the body of Christ in my properly clasped hands. I place the body in my mouth, *My body for your body.* I make the sign of the cross.

On the way to the priest, I realize Zee's behind, following me. Though she's not confirmed, though she's a Protestant, I decide she's as much of this place as me, filled with at least as much holy spirit. Quickly, I tell her to mime my hands.

What is the origin of the phrase "to fall ill"? It comes from the Latin *in morbum incidere.* Translating as "to fall sick," the actual origin of the phrase isn't entirely known, but the phrase is undeniably pre-Christian. A poet's logic goes like this: our angels, they fall to earth; our loved ones, they fall ill and enter the earth. But poetic logic is trumped by the body itself, removed from mythology: the ancient Greeks just called it like it was. When sick, bodies collapse. On the way back to our pew, Zee part of the parade, we pass the Stations of the Cross that portray Christ's body, falling in series, falling in marble, falling the third time, forever.

THE TRAVELLER IS PUZZLED BY THE IMPENETRABLE DARKNESS inside the room, for nothing is truly absolutely dark, especially on a winter's night with a full moon, light smashing against the snow. The traveller takes a step back, hoping to gain more perspective, and notices a slight reflection in the window. The figure behind the window remains perfectly concealed, although that he stands there is plain enough; the circumstance is strange. There is light, otherwise the traveller would not have safely ascended the stair; the light can be seen playing on the glass, creating a reflection, of what remains obscure; and though the interior of the room is utterly dark, the traveller knows he can see a shadow within, one directly opposite him. The traveller begins to think of the glass, of the window, of how the light so gently strikes it, of how it glimmers even in darkness. The traveller sees now the nature of his own reflection in the glass, of his own form previously obscure to him during the entire journey, for on that journey there was only snow and countless steps. In the glass, between himself and the shadow, the traveller sees that, all this time, he has been Burning Crown Jesus, flames glinting above a gleaming crown.

LETTER BURNT
ON THE CROWN

Burning Crown Jesus observes everyone on Earth. He's ready to listen, already listening, all knowing. His flames rise a little higher than before, probably because my despair is so intense.

BCJ, the cosmic loving force that wants everyone to cross the finish line, to get in from the cold, to make it to the church on time, doesn't intervene so much as encourage. He appears; he watches. I'm sure in other people's lives he sees success, presides over things like weddings and accolades and just being a good person. But in my life, he has to be there for me when I may die.

I think of suffering as an external thing, as if it were like a locomotive. Most of the time, it heads around or away. But sometimes I've tied myself to busy tracks, tired of a long journey, one that only leads to the past and suddenly snaps back to the present. There's nothing to say to BCJ. Well, maybe there is one thing.

"You seem angry to me, Burning Crown Jesus. Your flames consume your cross. Look—it's singed."

BCJ doesn't look. He has no need. He already knows. "This is the only way I can burn off the despair for you, Shane. Perhaps you don't understand, but sometimes I have to get angry to do the good things I need to do. And saving you is one of those things."

Once upon a time, I desperately desired an answer to the question "Will Kaz and Zee get better?" and "Is there a cure?" I wanted certain answers to be true. Yet not all stories are happy. Not everyone will be restored. That there was love, though—this account remains a love story.

As usual, BCJ's presence will have to suffice. That he cares has been the only constant good thing in my life. A bulwark. "Okay, Burning Crown Jesus," I say. And like that, things are good again. The flames on his head rise higher than I've ever seen. The flames seem constituted of delight, as if agitated by the wind, no longer embers thrown on my feelings. Finally, I realize: they are guardian flames.

HOSPITALS FIX NOTHING. They are to the modern era what churches used to be in the pre-modern: places where sacrifices are made, penalties received, cures attributed to divine intervention. Janet, Kaz, and I are back at McMaster's 2G clinic in the Yellow Zone. Yellow is nature's colour for danger—venom, caution. This is our shot at a second opinion.

Kaz remains tonic-clonic seizure-free, but Janet and I continue to be concerned. We both feel something is happening that has yet to be explained. We have yet to be listened to. What if there is something wrong that could be changed, helped? Kaz has frequent and excessive meltdowns, complains of seeing a "scary lady" at his window at night before falling asleep, and is behind his class because he cannot spell his name.

Dr. Green looks about my age. I watch this doctor very closely, as the parents of disabled children often do. Such parents want to know if their doctor is a People Who Care. In our special circumstance, we also want to know if Green is operating on bias forwarded by his colleague Cerulean, the holy fool who wouldn't order an MRI for my son, who wouldn't listen to our worry.

Dr. Green leans in very close, almost aggressively. "How can I help you today?" he says in a light South African accent. Maybe we are doomed and the bias has been forwarded. Is there no hope for Kaz?

"My son is sick. Perhaps you've heard?"

Janet speaks up: "We were referred to you by Dr. Cerulean. We had a disagreement with him and we're hoping someone can assume good care of Kaz."

Kaz marks the wall with a red crayon.

"Yes, well." Dr. Green says, and pauses, noticing Kaz's artistic choice of material.

"Kazzy, please use the paper," I say. "It's on the desk in front of you."

Kaz is in Grade One now, and his teacher does not want him because he is too much work. "He is still parallel-playing," she complains to us over the phone. "Do you think he even knows how far behind he is, that he's different?"

In the Yellow Zone, Kaz uses the paper sheet to make his red scribbles. He must interpret his splotches for me, I can never guess. "Bleedy poo!" he says, announcing the provenance of his masterpiece. "HAHAHAHA."

"Perhaps you can tell me the story again," Dr. Green says more softly. "I know you've had to tell it many times, but I'd appreciate it if you'd do so again. It might be helpful. I have read everything in Kaz's chart, but I still find it productive to hear from parents directly when we're starting out with one another."

We tell Kaz's story—from beginning to end. For the most part, the doctor doesn't interrupt. When he does, he asks for clarifications. He *listens*. I have elevated him provisionally to a Possible People Who Care.

When we finish, he gives us a medical explanation of Kaz based on our history. "I think it's Benign Rolandic Epilepsy," Dr. Green says, "based on what you've told me."

Dr. Green examines Kaz, cajoling and coaxing him through the exam. Eventually, a different resource nurse, Cream, returns with an EEG. "Ah!" Dr. Green says. "The EEG pattern fits, but there is also something else, something unexpected. Whenever Kaz falls asleep, he gets a massive increase in frontotemporal spikes. Areas of his brain are continuously spiking whenever he falls asleep. This makes it hard for him to learn, which fits with what you've said. It also makes it hard for him to get a good rest. The treatment for that is valproic acid, one of the medications he's already on. But there are other medications...." Case closed. I open the door to my heart and offer admittance to this People Who Care.

Who knows if the spikes were visible on Kaz's previous EEGs? Kaz experienced, every night for much of his life, a mounting form of permanent brain damage. Cerulean. Cerulean. Cerulean told us seizures happen, that some parents don't even bother to treat them, that their choice depends on their amount of worry. "It's up to you, your personal comfort level," he said. My own personal Jesus.

What I am curious about, looking back: did Cerulean miss a pattern of waves that marked Kaz as having an extremely rare form of epilepsy, making up only 0.5 percent of children with seizures? Were we not aggressive enough when treating Kaz because Cerulean didn't identify the monster in the wave pattern? Did Kaz go years unrecognized as having a monster under the bed?

We visit McMaster almost twenty more times to try to get the spikes under control—so many medication trials and failures. After a series of detailed neuropsychological tests conducted over three years, we learn that, indeed, Kaz has suffered brain damage. He has not grown cognitively.

When he was two and a half, I worried that he might die; I looked up at the sky and saw a child's mouth, blood flowing between the teeth; I saw legs, vibrating; I saw a tiny body falling as if it was shot, bang, then seize. The sky was a tormentor, a place where my worries projected and all the nightmares a parent could have played on loop. Even now, I avoid looking up, for fear of seeing the bloody gums, the bitten tongue, the collapsing body. But if the fear were more honest, the sky would not be a trauma portal at all, because my prayers to end the grand mal seizures were answered. Instead, it would be the darkness itself that would terrify me, for when Kaz's eyes closed at night, a thief was behind them, stealing what it could.

"Do you have any questions?" Dr. Green asks.

DEAR DR. CERULEAN,

I've thought about a lawsuit. I've even talked about a lawsuit with other doctors. They counsel me to go ahead, that the cost of care for my son due to the damage to his brain will be substantial. That damage—was it there, detectable from the very start, from the first moment we saw you, from the first EEG?

I haven't asked Dr. Green. I haven't requested the old charts. I haven't taken any of the necessary steps to indict your care other than, of course, to write this memoir about my son.

If the damage wasn't happening when we first met you, a special secret damage, then it did happen after, was happening after, was occurring after your team performed so poorly that I had to ask for care to occur elsewhere. But because I was angry, and because you are already a specialist, my son couldn't be seen by anyone who might otherwise have cared for him. The damage had its perfect playground.

Seizures are sticky. Have one, have more than one. Each additional seizure adds to the stickiness. My son has a rare, intractable seizure syndrome that you either didn't catch or that you neglected.

When the system fails, or people fall between the cracks, injuries compound.

Must I think of my son in terms of injury?

I must. You are to blame, and I shall carry my hatred of your lack of care forever. But no lawsuit, because going through this once almost killed me. I can't go through it again. As you and I both know, patients who press civil suits through the courts inevitably face exacerbations of their underlying conditions. Me, I'm worried that in taking you to court, that one day I'll jump off a building. Does this seem manipulative, this formulation? A no-win?

I hope not. All I wanted was for my son to be better. That's why I entrusted his care to you.

Sincerely,

Shane Neilson

"ARE YOU GOING TO SEND IT?" Burning Crown Jesus asks. He appears like the Christ of old from my childhood—long-haired, dressed in flowing thick golden robes, surrounded in a heavy brass frame. But then he steps out of the frame and, with his feet now on the ground, puts his hand on his hip, just like my daughter used to do. "Hmmmmph?"

"What do you think I should do?" I say. Maybe BCJ can make my decision for me. Maybe he can tip me off, let me know what the outcome will be, encourage me if it's a good one or dissuade me if bad.

"Hmmmmph," he repeats, then adds: "There are more things in heaven and earth than are dreamt of in your philosophy."

Okay. No insider trading then. No, wait. BCJ starts to bow, until the crown is at the level of my hand. A few inches more, and the paper would catch fire. I see. God is literally showing me the path by the light of his heavenly flame.

I place the single singed sheet on the hot tines and watch it ignite, curling on itself as if it is seized. A rotting into black, and then small blowing embers are agitated by Christ's own exhalations of air. I should have known. All these years, BCJ has long been expounding on this bit of Isaiah: *Behold, all ye that kindle a fire, that compass yourselves about with sparks: walk in the light of your fire, and in the sparks that ye have kindled.* "Shane, your children are the real reason you're here. I know you prefer to think of me for reasons of convenience and habit. Who, of course, would conjure a vision of their young daughter to discourse on death with? So you use me when you want to die but think of them only when you want to live. But man, I need a break. And you could use one too. The sparks you've kindled—compass yourself. Me, I've decided to do my Jesus thang on the big screen."

ENTER BURNING CROWN JESUS IS CANCELLED

I'm alone in the ambulance. Aren't we all alone in ambulances? I'm alone except for BCJ, of course. He is always with me.

Speed is discernible only by deceleration, a phenomenon felt inside the vehicle, or by witnessing passing landscape. There is no window inside the ambulance cabin, so I don't know how fast we're going. We could be hurtling to the end of the earth, or jogging to a local emergency—perhaps a child, who may be seizing.

BCJ wears paramedic gear. A siren—the sound is muffled in here, but outside I suspect the sound is deafening, nothing can ignore the signal. *ROOO ROOO.* A giant, soft, clumsy hand pushes us along. Soon the hand will be called to the table, or to come to the door to put snowpants on.

BCJ says something, but it's hard for me to make out. What is he saying? READ MY LIPS. NO NEW TAXES. No. ULTRA LOW PRICES. No. I'M SORRY. Yes. The Christ, the son of God, is apologizing.

Sorry for what? But then I know: my arms and legs are bound to a board. I cannot move.

BCJ bends down to my ear and says, "What's the meaning of life?" The question doesn't strike me as odd, coming from a God, one who seems to be genuinely seeking an answer, not quizzing me about my faith. BCJ seems to be searching himself, on a religious quest.

The ambulance wrenches to a dead stop. There's been an accident— we're a part of the accident. We must have hit whatever it is at blazing speed—if BCJ and I weren't secured with belts, we would have been thrown into the front wall. I wonder how the driver is doing?

"We must have hit a block," BCJ says, undoing his belt, getting ready to check on the driver and possibly save him.

"Wait," I say. I know there is no time for a full confessional, but I have to try. "The meaning is LIFE IS HARD AND THEN YOU DIE. No. YOU CAN'T TAKE IT WITH YOU WHEN YOU GO. No. I'M SORRY. Yes—the meaning of life is spending time with those you love, and generally failing to do so perfectly, even though perfection is a trick, a trap, or a paradox: for what else do they deserve?"

And with that, Jesus springs into action, leaping out the toy ambulance to save the three-year-old that just crashed us into a Lego tower. From the front of the ambulance I hear a dispatch radio saying that this will have to be a combo stop—next, we need to take the stairs and pick up a little girl. There's been a sadness like an accident and we need to save her too.

IN 2020, UNICEF PRODUCED A REPORT CARD evaluating how UN member nations were doing with regards to the health care of children. The report explained that France spent 3.68 percent of its GDP on child health and welfare. The UK spent 3.6 percent. I include these nations as a comparator to Canada for obvious reasons. Canada comes in at 1.6 percent. In terms of outcomes, we consequently rank 30th out of 38 evaluated developed nations with respect to physical health. Our rank in terms of mental health? 31st. Canada averages 9 suicides of adolescents per year per 100,000; France, 3.4; the UK, 3.7. At the time Kaz was experiencing medically refractory seizures, an expert panel recommended that Ontario's children should have universal access to "quality, evidence-based, comprehensive medical and surgical epilepsy care at the right time and the right place." The reason for this recommendation was the objectively terrible care patients were receiving. Ten years after the creation of an epilepsy network, would things be different now? Much has been reported on COVID-related backlogs in the socialized care system. In terms of kids with epilepsy, it has been reported that there have been difficulties for children to get access to medication and health care professionals because of the pandemic.

The joke I tell other parents with lived experience of disabled children goes like this: I pretend with them that I'm talking to a normie parent. I nod my head, acknowledging the disruptive behaviour of my son. "Yes, he is screaming. Yes, he is stomping and snorting. Uh-huh. I should show him some discipline, should I? I should teach him a lesson? Right. Listen, I have some advice to offer you right back. It could save your life, so listen carefully: Don't let your kids get sick." The fellow parent of a disabled child, we laugh 'til it hurts. For who can know until they are in our shoes? And who could actually stop the speeding train headed straight for their child?

A much reported-on phenomenon is the worsening of child mental health due to the pandemic. But Canada was doing poorly on that score already. I sometimes stare at my ceiling at night, noticing the stucco, counting the ridges, verifying their number, a technique to distract me from fantasizing about what it would have been like if COVID had occurred in the years 2010-2013, how my daughter might have fared. The joke I tell myself goes like this: "Aren't you glad COVID didn't happen then?" It hurts to laugh because I am glad. What would my family have done, if our disaster had moved ahead ten years? Would I be alive?

THE DISABLED SWIMMING CLASS has a pupil list of three. On the first day, a kid with thick scars showing on his lower spine, just above his swim trunks, needs to be coaxed into the pool by the leader and a team of green-shirted volunteers. I note the extreme atrophy of his legs: spina bifida? His hands stim wildly as he descends the small-angle ramp into the water and is led to a corner, where he stays until the end of the lesson. Another girl, maybe fourteen and also autistic based on expression and mild stimming, strides more boldly into the pool. She dodges past the volunteers and starts playing with a group of toddlers just one wall over in the kiddie section. She waves and talks at a little boy held protectively in his mother's arms. A volunteer encourages the girl to come back to the session, but it takes the booming voice of her father to get her to return. Her face shows instant terror as she races to where the other boy stands in the corner.

"I think you're supposed to go there, with them," I say to Kaz.

"They seem more disabled than me," he says.

"It all depends," I say.

Kaz smiles and waves at the leader, who nods to acknowledge that Kaz is part of the group. After a few minutes in the corner, Kaz gets sent to a different pool with two volunteers. Part of my vision is obscured by the pool; I can't see half his lane.

By this time the girl is walking the wall dividing the kid's pool from the Olympic-sized adult pool. She could fall and strike her skull open—the wall's wet. She reaches a basket of toys, which must have always been her object, and dumps out everything inside: pink flutter boards, toy watering cans, acrylic crocodiles, rubber duckies in a range of sizes. The objects immediately begin their mysterious journey according to Brownian motion, (x) embroiled in its plot to travel during a certain time interval (t) in water, whose coefficient of diffusion (D) is equal to half the average of the square of the displacement in the x-direction, somewhere between 1.2×10^{-6} to 6×10^{-6} cm^2/s. Her father is now at the water's edge, commanding her to stop, to go back with the instructors who are, like me, worried that she will fall.

Slipping into the pool, it's as if she remembers herself, somehow. She dips below the water and submerges for a second, but then pops back up, laughing. She drops down under the water and pops back up again. She's very willing to go back into the corner. The father retreats back to the bench beside me in the viewing area.

There, in the far end of the pool, Kaz comes into view. He's doing a choppy front crawl, and soon makes the wall and holds the edge, wiping the hair from his face. He smiles. Walking along the side of the pool the entire way are volunteers, cheering him on. They tell him something I cannot hear and he lets go of the wall. He doesn't sink. He must be treading water.

A thought scrapes by, dragging its nails on my mental chalkboard: *I hate my life.* But then it's gone.

Kaz. The mental touchstone, where is Kaz? He's no longer at the far end of the pool. The green volunteers are now approaching the shallow end, where I can see just a few feet at the extreme edge. Kaz's head pops into view, then his left arm completes a final stroke of the back crawl. Having reached the edge, he stops and holds on. The volunteers say something to him, I can't tell what, their backs are turned. Kaz laughs, says something back. Then they laugh, their backs heaving. And he's gone again as the volunteers spot him, walking slowly to the far end of the pool.

Did I ever think he'd be able to swim? There are so many 'did-I-ever's.' At two-and-a-half, the list long as milestones in a life, all the things Burning Crown Jesus is supposed to be there cheering for. Did I ever think he'd have a job? Did I ever think he'd fall in love with someone and have a relationship? Did I ever think he'd move out of my house? Did I ever think he'd be able to drive a car? No. I didn't. And he won't be able to do some of these, at least.

At the moment, he can swim. I want him to be able to understand units of time like an hour or half an hour, to know what money is and how much something costs. But right now, he's smiling. He's swimming. As sure as I am that my friend Burning Crown Jesus is real, I am certain that Kaz is happy.

"DAD, THERE ARE TOO MANY BACTERIA that I am supposed to know," Zee says. "This classification system is *wild*. Cocci, diplococci, bacilli? Gram-positive or gram-negative? Pathogenic or commensal? How do you keep all this information straight in your head?"

We drive in the middle lane of highway 401, my routine lane, my must-have. Being in the middle lane brings safety. We can't be shunted left or right because of unexpected, forced turning lanes. The middle lane always pours to the destination. Occupying the middle lane allows my mind to fret about things other than traffic and direction. Like: how is Zee?

"When you move on to actually practise medicine, the stuff they make you memorize becomes real diagnoses in real people. The body becomes your mnemonic. Everything you're learning now is abstract. Having symptoms to go on, clinical signs—these culminate in culture results.

Knowing how one arrives at the culture result, or working back from the result to the patient, makes remembering things a lot easier because it's more fun. And it's more fun because it's real."

"Ugh. I hate these lists of things. *Stupid* diplococci."

Something in the way she says this reminds me of her at ten years old, back when she was sick. Dyad is a synonym for two, something I learned when researching the topic of child suicide.

I'm moving Zee into her apartment in Toronto for her first year of medical school. The van is packed with clothes and small appliances. Every bit of space is occupied, except for the driver area. Zee is covered in bags on the passenger side.

"It will get easier," I say. "Look at me. Do you think I could do anything hard?"

Zee considers this. For most of her life, she's been the one to take instruction booklets from my hands and build an Ikea structure or hook up electronic devices. For some reason, a sequence of instructions eludes my understanding, especially when they involve spatial awareness. Put x here, turn y—mystifying. But Zee quickly completes such tasks. "Hmmmn. Maybe you're right!" she says, her laughter making the bags around her jostle.

I never pushed Zee to apply. I never wanted her to be a doctor, something I haven't told her. Besides, I want her to be herself—to be happy. Any warning I might offer would only come from a particular place and time. Zee isn't exactly like me. She's neurotypical. Beautiful. Resourceful. School won't do to her what it did to me because she won't go to school the way I did, the way I was.

"Can I forget most of it, though?" she asks, a pair of eyes and a mouth looking out from a pile of multicoloured bags.

I could answer the question systematically, responding that certain specialities, like internal medicine, depend upon information as their business; that family medicine is a kind of devolution from that lofty height, that some of the information must be retained and the general structure of it preserved, if not the specifics, so that the information can be reacquired quickly should a case come along; that each surgical speciality has its own unique domain of bugs particular to it; that even psychiatry must keep infection in the differential.

But I don't. "Today you can," I say, moving out of the middle lane and into the right, leaving the 401 for the 427.

THE INVITATION ARRIVED IN A FANCY GOLD ENVELOPE—*COME AND VISIT JERRY IN LOVELY STAMFORD, CONNECTICUT! HOTEL ACCOMMODATION AND AIRFARE ON US!* Then, dropping into lower case reasonableness: *We want to help you share your story with a worldwide daytime audience.*

Does the Nice Lady produce for NBC-Universal now? She tells me, "You know the show, right? We got moms who overfeed their babies. We got the paternity test reveals. Oh, and the cheaters. So, so many cheaters. We prefer the married cheaters, but we'll take just boyfriends and girlfriends, especially if there's a child involved. We have racists on from time to time, but since those episodes stress out security, we don't do them as often, and anyway, there's none today. Looks like just good 'ol infidelity and paternity, Shane. But I'll let you know if Jer changes things up." Despite what Nice Lady says, the green room is filled with midgets, strippers, and a legion of young men in white wifebeater tees. A little Pomeranian yaps at a man who is naked save for gauze bandages wrapped around his privates. Who knows who I'll be paired with? I gather they tape a run of five to six shows a day.

"Breaking the Sex Record!" yells Chuck Connors from somewhere. "Test, test. The Kung Fu Hillbilly! Mother Daughter Domination! Chopped Off His Own Manhood!" Well, at least I know why gauze man is here.

Nice Lady shoves me onstage. "Go get 'em, tiger!" she growls. So creepy. No, it's worse than that. I'm in an actual tiger suit. As my eyes meet the blazing studio lights, Chuck Conners says, "SO I MARRIED A FURRY." And every single audience member, all women, BOOOOO and HISSSSSS.

To my left, Burning Crown Jerry mock-chastises the audience. "Now now," he says. "Shane came all the way from Canada and maybe he's just in that suit because it's cold there, not because he has some kind of sexual hang-up involving tigers."

The audience, paid to hate and laugh, laughs. A microphone is passed to a particularly obese matron. "Hi. Faye from Minneapolis. Was there some kind of trauma that happened when you were young, perhaps when a fuzzy tiger stuffy was nearby, that caused you to develop this fixation?"

The audience goes crazy. "Go to *Oprah*! Go to *Oprah*!" The only person hated more than Faye is me. Time to go full WWE. I bend over and twerk for the crowd, heel-style, screaming "YOU KNOW YOU WANT SOME FURRY WURRY" even though I don't even know what a 'wurry' is. Wasn't I here to talk about my book? About how JESUS is R-E-A-L, and F-U-C-K Y-O-U if you don't believe, you heathen motherfuckers?

Jer has his security guards save Faye, who now sits with me on stage. Jer chuckles as he looks down at the ground and says, good-naturedly, "I have to ask. What does your wife think about all this?"

The audience hoots and hollers FAGGOT and FRUIT while Faye holds her hand over her heart whispering, "I'd nuzzle in your fuzzle anytime." Nuzzle in my fuzzle?

Faye, it seems, is already married. A man has burst into this live studio audience in a Pac-Man T-shirt and shouts, "Take your goddamned paws offa my wife!" My only hope is that the security guards can successfully repel his gelatinous onslaught. But before he can even come close, the audience taunts him. FATTY FATTY FATTY they chant about Faye, or him, or both, and Pac-Man is ready to take on the whole lot of them. Faye, though, loves the attention, and bares her breasts. "Where my Jerry Beads at?" she shouts in exultation.

Backstage, I hear an Ozarks accent say, "Is they callin' for me? The Kung Fu Hillbilly is ready, y'all!" But in the melee, I'm struck in the head. Before I collapse and soil my suit, I see Burning Crown Jerry off to the side, protected by Steve Wilkos. BCJ looks bemused, or is it pensive? Oh—he's about to Final Thought. Maybe I can hold on for just a minute more and hear.

The camera closes in on BCJ's face. "Well, it was a good show. We saw some skin—we even ran out of Jerry Beads!—and the fur flew. But I'm devoting this final thought to a different audience, to the folks at home. Some of you want to know if I am responsible for your immaculate conceptions. Apparently, many of you think I have visited in the night and left joy in your wombs. Well, last week Steve swabbed my cheek and we have the results back."

The studio speakers blare the bridge from Michael Jackson's Billie Jean. *Who. Who. Who. Who.* "I am sorry to report, I AM NOT the father!"

I let go to the faint strains of Billy Jean, feeling free to sink into thoughtlessness. Burning Crown Jesus is cancelled. For me, and because this is 2023. I'm going to have to make it to the end on my own, the love story has to be enough, see this through to the end.

BIBLIOGRAPHY

References to Texts

Bradbury, Ray. *The Martian Chronicles*. New York: Simon and Schuster. 2012.

Holy Bible, King James Version, The. New York: Oxford Edition. 1769.

Leenaars, A. (Ed.). *Lives and deaths: Selections from the works of Edwin S. Shneidman*. Philadelphia: Brunner/Mazel, 1999.

Nowlan, Alden. "It's Good to be Here." *Collected Poems of Alden Nowlan*. Fredericton: Goose Lane, 2017.

References to Popular Songs

Benny Andersson, Bjorn Ulvaeus, Stig Anderson. "Dancing Queen" from ABBA's *Arrival*. Polar Music. 1976.

William Bratton, composer. Jimmy Kennedy, lyrics. "Teddy Bear's Picnic." 1907.

Jacques Morali and Victor Willis. "Y.M.C.A." from the Village People's *Cruisin'*. 1978.

References to Television Programs

iCarly, created by Dan Schneider and airing in Canada on the YTV Network.

The 700 Club, currently hosted by Pat Robertson, airing in syndication in the United States of America for over fifty years.

The Cat in the Hat Knows a Lot About That, produced by Julie Stall and Helen Stroud, and based on the books by you know who.

Thomas & Friends, created by Britt Allcroft and produced by Gullane Entertainment (but based on the books by the Rev. W. Awdry and his son Christopher.

References to Web-Based Works

"The Duck Song" was written by Bryant Oden and is searchable on YouTube. The channel is ForrestFire Films.

DISCLAIMER

The chronology of the narrative line in *Saving* has been purposely simplified. Much happens in a life, let alone four lives, and I have smoothed out Kaz's seizure chronology in particular. The actual story is much worse than I have depicted. Conversations with health care staff captured in *Saving* are not verbatim. They are reconstructions from memory. In fact, the book itself is entirely a product of my memory, and this rendition of my memory tends towards the fantastical. In 'actual' existence are, it must be admitted, official notes written by doctors, nurses, and counsellors concerning the health of my children, but my creative record is as true as they are true. As the sign at the Silvercreek office of Trellis once said, "We are all able." As George Orwell would say about the sick children of Ontario, "All patients are equal, but some are more equal than others."

ACKNOWLEDGEMENTS

My thanks to the following publications that have printed work from the manuscript in its earlier incarnations:

Canadian Medical Association Journal
Journal of the American Medical Association
The Dalhousie Review
The Fiddlehead
The Medical Post
Riddle Fence

I thank the women at the Child Care and Learning Centre at the University of Guelph; Lorraine York, Grace Kehler, Luke Hill, and Jim Johnstone for reading this manuscript; hey, poetry!; and my immediate family most of all. Conor Kerr: no boats!